Available F
American Academ

Achieving a Healthy Weight for Your Child: An Action Plan for Families

ADHD: What Every Parent Needs to Know

Autism Spectrum Disorder: What Every Parent Needs to Know

Baby and Toddler Basics: Expert Answers to Parents' Top 150 Questions

Building Resilience in Children and Teens: Giving Kids Roots and Wings

Caring for Your Baby and Young Child: Birth to Age 5*

Caring for Your School-Age Child: Ages 5–12

Co-parenting Through Separation and Divorce: Putting Your Children First

Family Fit Plan: A 30-Day Wellness Transformation

Heading Home With Your Newborn: From Birth to Reality

My Child Is Sick! Expert Advice for Managing Common Illnesses and Injuries

New Mother's Guide to Breastfeeding

The New Baby Blueprint: Caring for You and Your Little One

Parenting Through Puberty: Mood Swings, Acne, and Growing Pains

The Picky Eater Project: 6 Weeks to Happier, Healthier Family Mealtimes

Raising an Organized Child: 5 Steps to Boost Independence, Ease Frustration, and Promote Confidence

Raising Kids to Thrive: Balancing Love With Expectations and Protection With Trust

Retro Baby: Cut Back on All the Gear and Boost Your Baby's Development With More Than 100 Time-tested Activities

Retro Toddler: More Than 100 Old-School Activities to Boost Development

For additional parenting resources, visit the HealthyChildren bookstore at https://shop.aap.org/for-parents.

*This book is also available in Spanish.

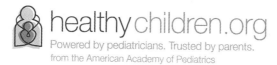

Foreword by *New York Times* notable author Mona Hanna-Attisha, MD, MPH, FAAP

Protecting Your Child's Health

EXPERT ANSWERS TO URGENT **ENVIRONMENTAL** QUESTIONS

Ruth A. Etzel, MD, PhD, FAAP
Editor in Chief

Sophie J. Balk, MD, FAAP
Associate Editor

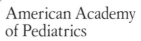

American Academy
of Pediatrics

DEDICATED TO THE HEALTH OF ALL CHILDREN®

American Academy of Pediatrics Publishing Staff

Mary Lou White, *Chief Product and Services Officer/SVP, Membership, Marketing, and Publishing*
Mark Grimes, *Vice President, Publishing*
Holly Kaminski, *Editor, Consumer Publishing*
Shannan Martin, *Production Manager, Consumer Publications*
Amanda Helmholz, *Medical Copy Editor*
Peg Mulcahy, *Manager, Art Direction and Production*
Sara Hoerdeman, *Marketing Manager, Consumer Products*

Published by the American Academy of Pediatrics
345 Park Blvd
Itasca, IL 60143
Telephone: 630/626-6000
Facsimile: 847/434-8000
www.aap.org

The American Academy of Pediatrics is an organization of 67,000 primary care pediatricians, pediatric medical subspecialists, and pediatric surgical specialists dedicated to the health, safety, and well-being of all infants, children, adolescents, and young adults.

The information contained in this publication should not be used as a substitute for the medical care and advice of your pediatrician. There may be variations in treatment that your pediatrician may recommend based on individual facts and circumstances.

Statements and opinions expressed are those of the authors and not necessarily those of the American Academy of Pediatrics.

Any websites, brand names, products, or manufacturers are mentioned for informational and identification purposes only and do not imply an endorsement by the American Academy of Pediatrics (AAP). The AAP is not responsible for the content of external resources. Information was current at the time of publication.

The persons whose photographs are depicted in this publication are professional models. They have no relation to the issues discussed. Any characters they are portraying are fictional.

The publishers have made every effort to trace the copyright holders for borrowed materials. If they have inadvertently overlooked any, they will be pleased to make the necessary arrangements at the first opportunity.

This publication has been developed by the American Academy of Pediatrics. The contributors are expert authorities in the field of pediatrics. No commercial involvement of any kind has been solicited or accepted in the development of the content of this publication. Disclosures: All contributors discussed no relevant financial relationships.

Every effort has been made to ensure that the drug selection and dosages set forth in this publication are in accordance with the current recommendations and practice at the time of publication. It is the responsibility of the health care professional to check the package insert of each drug for any change in indications or dosage and for added warnings and precautions.

Every effort is made to keep *Protecting Your Child's Health: Expert Answers to Urgent Environmental Questions* consistent with the most recent advice and information available from the American Academy of Pediatrics.

Special discounts are available for bulk purchases of this publication. Email Special Sales at nationalaccounts@aap.org for more information.

Printed in the United States of America

9-453/0920   1 2 3 4 5 6 7 8 9 10
CB0121
ISBN: 978-1-61002-437-2
eBook: 978-1-61002-438-9
EPUB: 978-1-61002-439-6
Mobi: 978-1-61002-440-2

Library of Congress Control Number: 2020937623

What People Are Saying About *Protecting Your Child's Health*

"The first-time parent faces a bewildering array of products and recommendations. In *Protecting Your Child's Health*, Drs Etzel and Balk cut through the thicket of research and received wisdom to provide parents with informed analysis and practical advice. This is the only baby book you will ever need to understand how to best protect your child from environmental hazards."
—Stephanie M. Chalupka, EdD, RN, PHCNS-BC, professor and director, master of science in nursing program, Worcester State University

"Exactly the type of information parents need to know. Finally, a book with clear and actionable information for parents. The Q&A format makes it easy for parents to get real answers. Sound science, practical and precautionary advice, and a healthy dose of heart. Parents have deserved this for a long time; this book is a tool for parental empowerment."
—Patricia Butterfield, PhD, RN, FAAN, professor, Elson S. Floyd College of Medicine, and dean emerita of nursing, Washington State University

"There has never been a more appropriate time for the release of this important work focused on protecting the health of our children. Ruth Etzel has always been and continues to be the voice of the millions of children on our planet who need the protections described in this work."
—Linda McCauley, RN, PhD, FAAN, dean and professor, Nell Hodgson Woodruff School of Nursing, Emory University

"Dr Etzel has been a quiet warrior and fierce advocate for the protection of children's health for decades. Her amazing new book equips parents with critical tools to combat the myriad of environmental health threats that families, often unknowingly, face every day. By using the information provided, parents will be far more empowered to help ensure better health outcomes and lifelong opportunities for their children."
—Ruth Ann Norton, president and CEO, Green & Healthy Homes Initiative

"It's so refreshing to have a down-to-earth pediatrician give practical advice to help parents understand the environmental risks their families face. I thank my lucky stars that Dr Etzel, through this book and her lifetime of work, empowers parents like me to advocate for our kids' health. It's groundbreaking to have a pediatrician encourage parents to raise their voices to confront transportation challenges, climate change, and the prospect of oil and gas wells in their neighborhoods."

—Elizabeth Brandt, MSW, Moms Clean Air Force

Editors

Editor in Chief
Ruth A. Etzel, MD, PhD, FAAP
Adjunct Professor
Milken Institute School of Public Health
The George Washington University
Washington, DC

Associate Editor
Sophie J. Balk, MD, FAAP
Attending Pediatrician
The Children's Hospital at Montefiore
Professor of Pediatrics
Albert Einstein College of Medicine
Bronx, NY

Contents

Foreword

In the summer of 2015, a 4-month-old named Nakala came to the pediatric clinic with her mom for a checkup. Like all pediatricians, I followed the usual routine: We look in ears, noses, and throats. We listen to hearts, lungs, and tummies. We make sure kids are eating well, growing, and developing. We vaccinate them to protect them from bad diseases. And most importantly, we try our best to listen to parents and answer their questions.

So much of our privileged work as pediatricians is not as much about caring for the child in front of us today (although we love doing that) as it is about making sure children have the healthiest and brightest future possible. Our work is nestled in prevention and promise.

At that clinic visit, Nakala's mom said that she wanted to stop breastfeeding. I shared the many benefits of breast-feeding and urged her to continue. She had to go back to work, she said, and pumping was near impossible as a waitress. She planned to switch to powdered formula mixed with water but had some concerns. "Is the water all right?" she, looking skeptical, asked me. *"I heard things."*

The water. I'd been asked about it before. It had been over a year since Flint's water source had been changed from the Great Lakes to the local Flint River to save money. Although there were concerns in the local media about color, odor, taste, and even bacteria in the water, they were always met with repeated reassurances by multiple levels of government—by officials and experts charged with keeping us, especially our children, healthy and safe.

Standing there, with my white coat and doctor's confidence, I nodded without hesitation. "The tap water is just fine," I told Nakala's mom.

But I was wrong about that. Despite years of medical training and a background in environmental health, I had been blinded. And, perhaps even worse, I had failed at Pediatrics 101, the underlying and unwritten philosophy in my profession that *moms are always right*. Dads and other caregivers are too, of course.

By now you know that the water in Flint was not "just fine." The severely corrosive Flint water was not being treated properly; it had been leaching lead from our old pipes and lead had been going straight into our drinking water. The lead levels in our water were in the thousands and thousands of parts per billion (that's a lot; the US Environmental Protection Agency has set a goal of zero for the maximum contaminant level of lead in water).

When I heard about the possibility of lead in the water, my life changed. I thought about Nakala and the thousands of other Flint kids just like her. As a pediatrician, I literally took an oath to care for and protect kids. That is what drove me to conduct research that showed that lead wasn't just in the drinking water; it was in the bodies and blood of Flint kids. And along with a growing and unexpected team—moms, dads, pastors, activists, students, scientists, journalists, and doctors—we finally got the government to take action. Since then, we have been building a model of recovery and promise for our kids and we are hoping that the lessons we learn will help children everywhere. And above all, the most important concept to share is that of prevention.

Fortunately, this new book from the American Academy of Pediatrics addresses many aspects of prevention. It helps answer important questions that you may have about environmental exposures your child may face and how to prevent or lessen those exposures. It covers a wide variety of topics that parents have asked pediatricians all over the country about. It provides practical information to help build the best possible future for your child.

As you read this book, remember the story of Flint and the untapped superpower you—as parents, grandparents and other caregivers—have to prevent exposures by making the environments where our children live safer and healthier. For some of us, that power means making more informed individual decisions for your own children, such as what food to eat and the products to buy. But remember, your superpower also gives you the opportunity to fight for all the kids in a school, a neighborhood, a city, a state, and even a country. Your actions, such as getting more informed by reading this book or raising your voice, asking questions, holding leaders and industries accountable, fighting for science and prevention-based policies, and voting, can make a tremendous difference in the lives of not just one child, like Nakala, but countless children who need care and protection.

And if we work collectively together, we ensure a safe environment and a healthy future for generations to come.

Dr Hanna-Attisha
New York Times notable author of *What The Eyes Don't See: A Story of Crisis, Resistance, and Hope in an American City*

Preface

In the mid-1990s, the American Academy of Pediatrics (AAP) realized that pediatricians needed more information about the effects of the environment on the health of children who pediatricians take care of. Pediatricians needed to know more about key environmental issues, such as molds in the home, mercury in fish, ozone in the air, and the many other chemicals in the environment, to best advise parents. At that time, information for pediatricians was scattered in different places and there were no books with information all in one place. The AAP sought to fill that void by publishing *Pediatric Environmental Health,* the first-ever handbook on environmental health geared toward pediatricians. Since that time, as information about pediatric environmental health has greatly expanded, the AAP has published 3 more editions, with the fourth edition of *Pediatric Environmental Health* released in 2019. In each edition, every chapter includes frequently asked questions (FAQs)—questions to which parents need answers. The FAQs of the fourth edition are the basis of this book for parents, *Protecting Your Child's Health: Expert Answers to Urgent Environmental Questions.*

We have had the privilege of being the editors of all the editions. Every edition contains many chapters, each written by an individual author. As editors, we have worked with dozens of authors, including 72 who wrote chapters for the fourth edition. The authors are pediatricians and scientists who are experts in their specific areas of pediatric environmental health. We are greatly indebted to each and every author who volunteered to write an up-to-date chapter, including these important FAQs. We also thank the members of the AAP Council on Environmental Health Executive Committee for their review of chapters in each edition of the handbook. We specifically thank Paul Spire, who staffs the AAP Council on Environmental Health, for his ongoing commitment in promoting pediatric environmental health.

We owe a special debt of gratitude to Jeff Mahony, senior director of professional and consumer publishing at the AAP, and Holly Kaminski, editor of consumer publishing at the AAP, for their vision in having the book created and for their incredible commitment to getting it into the hands of parents who can benefit from it. We also appreciate the excellent work of Amanda Helmholz, the copy editor.

To the parents who will read this book: you have the most important job in the world as guardians of your children. We are committed to working in partnership with you to ensure that their futures are as bright, healthy, and safe as possible.

Ruth A. Etzel, MD, PhD, FAAP
Sophie J. Balk, MD, FAAP

Introduction

As pediatricians who care for infants, children, and adolescents, we know that hardly a week goes by during which parents don't hear a story or read a blog about the effects of the environment on children's health. In 2020 the pandemic of COVID-19 swept across the world and showed that health and the environment are very much intertwined. Spread from person to person by coughing, breathing, and talking with others nearby, it clearly demonstrated the risks of living and working close to other people. During the previous year, stories about the disastrous fires in Australia showed the total impact, over the years, of slowly increasing climate change on the continent. Dramatic events such as these offer an opportunity to focus on children's environmental health issues, to teach children about them, and to bring attention to the importance of prevention. They also highlight the many different "environments" in which a child lives: the bedroom, the home, the school, the neighborhood, the park, the community, the state, the country, the world—these are circles, each one larger than the next. Although large-scale events such as massive forest fires heighten our awareness that environmental crises have important physical and psychological effects on children and their families, it is easy to overlook the fact that less visible (or invisible) environmental threats can also have important physical and psychological effects. We must pay attention to the highly visible threats and the invisible threats to infants, children, and adolescents. It is especially important to focus on our young people because compared with adults, children are often more susceptible to environmental health hazards. We must also focus on the many positive aspects of the environment, such as being outside in nature.

This book is composed of frequently asked questions from the fourth edition of *Pediatric Environmental Health*, a handbook for pediatricians published by the American Academy of Pediatrics. This new book, *Protecting Your Child's Health: Expert Answers to Urgent Environmental Questions*, provides a foundation for learning more about environmental health. The book is intended for you: the parents and other caregivers of children, as well as others, interested in preventing children's exposures to environmental hazards during infancy, childhood, and adolescence. You may be looking for guidance about how to evaluate news reports about possible hazards in the air, water, and food. Sometimes, scientists and researchers don't yet have all the information needed to have a definitive answer about the effects of a chemical hazard. In those situations, what do pediatricians advise parents to do? There are often no easy answers to questions about an environmental hazard. Each possibly hazardous exposure must be considered in light of other problems facing the child and of social, financial, emotional, and intellectual resources available to confront them. After fully understanding the facts and what scientists know and do not know, different parents may choose different ways to respond to the scientific information we do have.

The goal of this book is to provide parents with practical answers to questions about specific pollutants and situations that are encountered in daily life. We hope that the information will foster a better understanding of how important it is for children to live in a healthy environment. We aim to illustrate ways to promote healthy environments for children.

We also want to make readers aware of the controversial areas and gaps in scientific information. Knowledge about the impact of the environment on children's health has been growing very fast for the past 20 years. New information is being discovered, and our understanding of existing information is constantly being updated and expanded. As the fields of environmental health and medicine evolve, what pediatricians recommend to you may change with the publication of additional findings. Armed with the information in this book, every family can try to take steps to prevent unnecessary exposures in their own home, child care setting, and school. History shows that individual parents have been responsible for major changes in improving children's environments. For example, a single family in Michigan with a child poisoned by mercury helped change national policy on the use of mercury as a preservative in paint. So don't be afraid to jump in and get involved. While you are increasing your knowledge about the impact of contaminants on child health, it may be helpful to work with other parents in your community. Also, several national organizations such as those listed in the Resources section of the Appendix offer opportunities for involvement. A first step might be to get involved at your child's school, or to teach your child the importance of recycling. You can start small by making some changes in the items that you purchase for cleaning your home and by encouraging your children to understand what you are doing and to follow in your footsteps. Getting your kids and the family to be outside in nature is good for everyone's physical and mental health. It is also important to advocate for policies in your community and at the state and national levels that ensure clean air, water, and food and a livable planet for future generations. See the Resources section of the Appendix for ideas about ways to be involved. The next generation will benefit from your actions today.

Chapter 1

A Healthy Family Begins Before the Baby Arrives

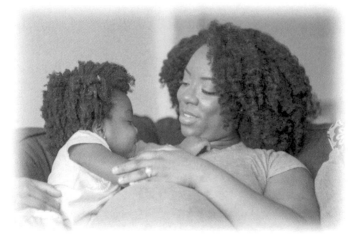

1. **What can I do before I become pregnant to ensure the healthiest possible pregnancy and to reduce the chance that my baby will have a birth defect?**

Schedule a preconception visit with your doctor (or other clinician). Preconception health care is care that a woman of childbearing age receives before pregnancy. A preconception visit can help you and your doctor to identify and treat health conditions that may cause problems during your pregnancy. These conditions include high blood pressure, diabetes mellitus, seizure disorders, and certain infections. The visit gives your clinician the opportunity to discuss important subjects such as nutrition, weight, exercise, stress reduction, smoking cessation and secondhand smoke exposure, avoiding alcohol, avoiding fish high in levels of mercury, and avoiding recreational and occupational exposures that may pose risks. This is also an opportunity for your clinician to administer any missing vaccines and to make adjustments to any medications you are taking to ensure that they are the safest possible.

In addition to asking about your health history, your clinician will ask about your partner's and family's health. If you or your partner have a history of birth defects or premature births, or if either of you has a high risk for a genetic disorder on the basis of family history, ethnic background, or age, your clinician may suggest that you see a genetic counselor.

Any woman of childbearing age should take a folic acid supplement every day. Ingesting 0.4 milligrams (mg) of folic acid every day will prevent certain kinds of birth defects, particularly defects of the nervous system. Pregnant women should increase their folic acid intake to 0.6 mg per day. Folic acid should be taken by all women of childbearing age because many pregnancies are not planned and women may not know they are pregnant until the first trimester is well under way. Folic acid is available as part of many multivitamin supplements.

2. **What can I do while I'm pregnant to improve the likelihood of having a healthy, full-term baby?**

The first step in having a healthy baby is ensuring that the mother is healthy.

Iodine is a mineral found in some foods. Iodine is needed to make thyroid hormones. Iodine supplementation is important because iodine deficiency occurs to some extent in about one-third of pregnant women in the United States. This deficiency may be worsened by environmental exposures. For example, perchlorate (a common contaminant in food and water) prevents normal hormone production in the thyroid. This means that iodine levels are reduced and also affects the normal levels of iodine in breast milk. Women should take prenatal vitamin supplements that include at least 150 micrograms of iodine. Women also should use iodized salt to help maintain an adequate iodine intake.

Make sure that any medications you take are safe to use during pregnancy. Do not drink alcohol, do not smoke tobacco or use electronic cigarettes, and try to avoid others who smoke. Avoid eating the 4 large, predatory fish that contain high amounts of mercury (swordfish, shark, tilefish, and king mackerel) and limit your intake of white (albacore) tuna. It is important to continue to regularly eat (at least two 3-ounce servings a week) other seafood before and during pregnancy, especially seafood rich in fatty acids and low in levels of mercury (such as salmon, pollock, or scallops) to ensure that sufficient amounts of the essential fatty acids docosahexaenoic acid (for short, DHA) and eicosapentaenoic acid (for short, EPA) are available for the development of the fetal brain.

If you work with chemicals, become informed about the possible risks those chemicals could pose to your fetus and take necessary precautions. Remember that environmental hazards can exist not only at work but also at home or even as a result of other household members' exposures. Be aware of potential environmental exposures that might occur during preparation for the baby's arrival such as remodeling the nursery—renovation could possibly result in lead exposure from removing lead-based paint.

Editors' note: Many of the issues that affect health and that are covered in the rest of this book count for two—a woman and her baby—when a woman is pregnant. Be sure to review the answers to other questions in this book to help you make decisions for both you and your baby.

3. **Is there any information about chemical exposures and risks to women who work in hair or nail salons?**

Working at nail and hair salons involves several chemicals. Hair salons may use chemicals such as aromatic amines (hair dye) or formaldehyde-based disinfectants. Nail salons use solvents, such as acetone or toluene, and acrylates. Because there are multiple substances and differences in ventilation and time of exposure, the reproductive health risks are difficult to determine.

Very few human studies examine multiple substance exposures and associated health risks. Hairdressers should have a work environment that includes wearing gloves, avoiding standing for long periods of time, ensuring good ventilation, covering products and garbage when they are not in use, and maintaining separate areas to eat.

Nail salons have similar issues. Nail salon workers should have good ventilation, keep products and garbage closed if they are not in use, remove garbage frequently, use appropriate dust masks for grinding nails, use gloves, and have a separate place to eat.

Avoid products (such as some types of acrylic nails) containing liquid methyl methacrylate (MMA) because studies of animals exposed to MMA show harm to the respiratory tract and liver. Information about protecting nail salon workers may be found at the Nail Salon Project of the US Environmental Protection Agency (www.epa.gov/saferchoice/protecting-health-nail-salon-workers-0).

4. **My partner and I are planning to adopt a child from outside of the United States. How can I find information about environmental exposures to which the adopted child may have been exposed?**

Because exposure to lead and lead poisoning are more common in other nations, you may want to ask your child's doctor to obtain a sample of the child's blood to determine the lead level. Other exposures depend on the country of origin. Consult with an expert from the Pediatric Environmental Health Specialty Units (www.pehsu.net), or an expert in adoption, to determine any next steps.

5. **What are the concerns about cell phone use among pregnant women?**

Three studies on this topic from the Danish National Birth Cohort have been published. Two studies demonstrated that cell phone use during pregnancy was associated with behavioral difficulties in the child, such as emotional and hyperactivity problems, around the age of school entry. A third study of cell phone use during pregnancy did not identify delays in development among children up to 18 months of age. Additional research from other populations is needed to clarify this issue.

6. **Should pregnant women, lactating women, or women planning pregnancy avoid eating fish?**

No known risk outweighs the benefit of eating seafood and fish. Both are sources of high-quality protein and beneficial omega-3 fatty acids. Current recommendations for pregnant women and young children include

- Eat 8 to 12 ounces (2–3 servings) of a variety of fish a week.

- Choose fish lower in levels of mercury, such as salmon, shrimp, pollock, tuna (light, canned), tilapia, catfish, and cod. Limit your intake of white (albacore) tuna.

- Avoid tilefish from the Gulf of Mexico, shark, swordfish, and king mackerel because they have the highest mercury levels.

- If you eat fish caught from streams, rivers, and lakes, pay attention for fish advisories on those water bodies.

Scientific studies show that the beneficial effects of breastfeeding outweigh any potential effects on a baby's development that could be due to the presence of contaminants (such as mercury) in human milk.

7. I am pregnant and live in a building that is old; I am worried about lead. Will it affect my baby?

If you have an elevated lead level, it could harm your baby. It is a good idea to get your blood lead level checked. If it is high, then you should find out whether there is lead in the paint or some other source, such as tap water. Once the source is identified, you should either have the lead removed or find a way to move out of harm's way. If you are worried, you should contact the Poison Control Center at 1-800-222-1222, the regional US Environmental Protection Agency office (www.epa.gov//aboutepa/visiting-regional-office), or the Pediatric Environmental Health Specialty Units (www.pehsu.net).

8. I did not know I was pregnant and went to a wedding where I had champagne and where people were smoking. I am worried that the champagne and the smoke will harm my baby. What should I do?

It is appropriate that you are concerned about these risks to your baby. To clearly and accurately evaluate the risks of each of those exposures, it is important that you see an obstetrician as soon as possible to discuss your concerns and to receive good prenatal care and close monitoring of your pregnancy. These actions go a long way toward reducing risks and ensuring a promising positive outcome.

Chapter 2

Feeding Your Baby

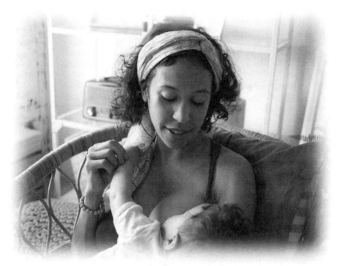

Editors' note: Breastfeeding provides ideal nutrition for the healthy growth and development of babies. Questions sometimes arise, however, about chemicals that may be transmitted to the baby from breast milk. Some of these questions are in this chapter. The benefits of breastfeeding greatly outweigh the potential risks in nearly every circumstance, and the American Academy of Pediatrics continues to strongly recommend breastfeeding.

Breastfeeding

1. Should I stop breastfeeding because I have been exposed to a chemical that can get into breast milk?

Breastfeeding provides well-known advantages for infants and mothers, as well as to families and society. The benefits of breastfeeding (especially prolonged breastfeeding) for the baby are a stronger immune system, fewer illnesses including ear infections, a lower chance of obesity, a lower chance of childhood cancer, and better brain development.

A number of environmental pollutants can cross from the mother into her breast milk, but breastfeeding need not be avoided or discontinued unless a dramatic exposure to the mother has occurred (such as a large unintentional chemical spill that is nearby). Breastfeeding may counter the subtle harms associated with a background level exposure to some common chemicals that a baby in the womb experiences.

2. Should I get my breast milk tested for chemical pollutants?

No. Traces of many chemicals can be found in breast milk; measuring them is difficult, and there are no programs to promote the quality of this testing. Even if a very good laboratory provides results, there are no accepted normal or safe values with which to compare. The benefits of breastfeeding far outweigh any risks posed by most chemical contaminants.

3. **Could my child's illness be caused by a contaminant in my breast milk?**

Nursing infants have been poisoned by contaminant chemicals in human milk, although in most cases, the mother herself was also ill. This phenomenon is extraordinarily rare.

4. **If I lose weight while I am breastfeeding, will that increase the levels of contaminants in my body because the same amount of contaminants will be dissolved in a smaller amount of fat? If I lose weight, will that lead to the contaminants coming out of fat and allow their levels to increase in my breast milk?**

No one has measured the levels of chemicals in human milk during weight loss. The greatest reported average weight loss among women who breastfeed in the long term is 9.7 pounds (lb) at 1 year, compared with a 5.3-lb loss in non-breastfeeding women. Other studies show little or no weight loss among breast-feeding women.

Breastfeeding women who are overweight and exercise and restrict calories can achieve weight loss faster and lose it mostly as fat. Theoretically, because the same amount of chemical would be stored in 9.7 lb less of tissue, mostly fat, weight loss might increase the concentration of the fat-soluble contaminants by up to 25%.

Breastfeeding does decrease the amount of contaminants in a mother's body. The concentration per unit of milk would be higher if the mother had lost body fat, but there should be no "mobilization" beyond that. Little evidence exists that shows that background exposure to contaminated human milk produces any ill consequences in children. Conversely, there is reasonable evidence that obesity in the mother does have consequences. Therefore, it is reasonable for a woman to follow a sensible diet and to exercise while she is breastfeeding her baby.

5. If I smoke, can I breastfeed?

Human milk is ideal for infants, regardless of whether a mother smokes. However, breastfeeding mothers should stop smoking. Nicotine, thiocyanate, and other toxicants are transferred through human milk to the infant. Another reason not to smoke and breastfeed is that infants of women who smoke stop breastfeeding at an earlier age. If a mother does continue to smoke, she should never breastfeed and smoke at the same time because a high concentration of smoke will be close to the infant. It is also advised not to smoke immediately before breastfeeding.

Breastfeeding women should not use electronic cigarettes. In addition, smoking or vaping any tobacco product, including vaping electronic cigarettes, should be banned inside the home or vehicle.

6. I live 30 miles (48 kilometers) from a nuclear reactor. Should I still breastfeed my baby if there is a meltdown?

Radioiodine from a nuclear meltdown is secreted into human milk. If a nuclear meltdown occurs, women who are breastfeeding should immediately contact the local health department to be given a medicine called potassium iodide (KI). This medicine should be given to the mother and the infant within 4 hours of the radiation contamination. A mother can continue to breastfeed her infant when the risk of exposure to radioiodine is temporary and if appropriate KI doses are given to the mother and infant within 4 hours of the radiation contamination. If this is not the situation, the mother and infant should receive priority for protective measures, such as evacuation.

Breastfeeding mothers should consider temporarily stopping breastfeeding and switching to either expressed milk (that was pumped and stored before the radiation exposure) or ready-to-feed infant formula until the mother can be seen by a doctor for appropriate treatment with KI. If no other source of food is available for the infant, the mother should continue to breastfeed, after washing the nipple and breast thoroughly with soap and warm water and gently wiping around and away from the infant's mouth.

7. **Should women who have been treated with radioiodine breastfeed?**

No. Breastfeeding is inadvisable for a woman who is being treated with radioiodine. Mothers should not resume breastfeeding for the current child after receiving radioiodine treatment but may safely breastfeed babies they may have in the future.

8. **I've learned that my drinking water was contaminated with perfluoroalkylated and polyfluoroalkylated substances (PFAS). Should I stop breastfeeding my infant?**

Even though a number of environmental pollutants such as perfluoroalkylated and polyfluoroalkylated substances (PFAS) can readily pass to the infant through human milk, the advantages of breastfeeding continue to outweigh potential risks in nearly every circumstance. The American Academy of Pediatrics and other organizations recommend continuing to breastfeed. Using bottled water for drinking can reduce further exposure.

9. **Because human milk can contain flame retardants such as polybrominated diphenyl ethers (PBDEs), should I stop breastfeeding my infant?**

Breastfeeding is recommended for infants. Numerous research studies have documented the many important advantages for infants, mothers, families, and society related to breastfeeding. Some of these benefits include immunologic advantages, lower obesity rates, and better brain development for the infant in addition to health advantages for the lactating mother. Even though a number of environmental pollutants, including flame retardants such as polybrominated diphenyl ethers (PBDEs), can readily pass to the infant through human milk, the advantages of breastfeeding outweigh potential risks in nearly every circumstance. The American Academy of Pediatrics and other organizations recommend breastfeeding.

10. **Given that persistent organic pollutants (POPs) are known to concentrate in human milk, is it safe for women who have eaten large quantities of game fish to breastfeed their infants?**

Authoritative bodies that have studied the safety of breastfeeding, including the American Academy of Pediatrics and the World Health Organization, have concluded that the benefits of breastfeeding outweigh any risks from exposures to persistent organic pollutants (POPs) or toxic chemicals in human milk. Breastfeeding, especially prolonged breastfeeding, conveys enormous health and psychological benefits to the child including greater resistance to infections and a reduced risk of childhood cancer.

11. Will breastfeeding reduce my baby's exposure to chemicals that leach from plastic bottles or formula can linings, including bisphenol A (BPA)?

Bisphenol A (BPA) is a chemical that leaches from some plastic bottles or formula can linings. Although low concentrations of BPA have been detected in human milk, breastfeeding a baby is one way to reduce exposure to this chemical. The American Academy of Pediatrics recommends exclusive breast-feeding for a minimum of 4 months but preferably for 6 months. Breastfeeding should be continued, with the addition of complementary foods, at least through the first 12 months of age and thereafter as long as mutually desired by the mother and infant.

12. What are safe nipple emollients to use during breastfeeding?

Purified lanolin is commonly used and is safe for mother and baby. Plant-based oils can also be safe options, and human milk itself can be used to soothe and soften sore nipples.

13. How should human milk be stored and heated?

Human milk can be stored at room temperature for 4 hours, in the refrigerator for 3 days, and in the freezer for 9 months. Human milk should be heated by placing the filled bottle in a warm container or pot. It is important not to submerge the bottle. Always test the milk on the inside of the wrist to make sure it is not too hot to give to your baby.

Bottle-feeding and Formula

14. What is the recommended way to prepare infant formula?

Water used for mixing infant formula must be from a safe water source, as defined by the state or local health department. If you are concerned or uncertain about the safety of tap water, you may use bottled water or bring cold tap water to a rolling boil for 1 minute (no longer), then cool the water to room temperature for no more than 30 minutes before it is used. Warmed water should be tested in advance to make sure it is not too hot for the infant. The easiest way to test the temperature is to shake a few drops on the inside of the wrist.

Otherwise, a bottle can be prepared by adding powdered formula and room temperature water from the tap just before feeding. Bottles made in this way from powdered formula can be ready for feeding because no additional refrigeration or warming is required.

Prepared formula must be discarded within 1 hour after serving it to an infant. Prepared formula that has not been given to an infant may be stored in the refrigerator for 24 hours to prevent bacterial contamination.

15. Can my daughter switch to soy formula because she has lactose intolerance? Will isoflavones in soy formula cause harmful effects in her?

It is very unusual for an infant to be born with lactose intolerance. Lactose intolerance, if it develops, usually occurs later in childhood. Nevertheless, many infants are given soy infant formula (made from soybeans) because soy protein–based formula is lactose-free.

Lactose-free and reduced-lactose cow milk–based formulas are also available. Soy formula contains much higher levels of isoflavones (chemical compounds in soy that have hormonal activity) than does human milk or cow milk–based formula. Experimental studies of animals have shown that high-level genistein (one compound in the isoflavone category) can cause harmful effects to reproduction and development. Studies using soy infant formula in experimental animals were not conclusive. Currently, there are some data on the effects of isoflavone exposure in human infants who were fed soy formula. More research is needed in this area.

16. **Are the phytoestrogens in soy formula related to early puberty?**

Soy infant formula contains phytoestrogens (plant-based estrogens) that are weak estrogenic compounds. Isoflavones in soy formula have estrogenic effects that are probably orders of magnitude lower than those of estradiol, the natural human estrogen. There is one report of soy infant formula use and premature breast development in girls younger than 2 years. Early puberty in girls younger than 8 years or boys younger than 9 years may be caused by hormone exposure from outside the body.

17. **Is it possible to reduce isoflavone levels in soy infant formula?**

Isoflavone levels vary in soybeans depending on geographic location and weather conditions. This variation can probably be used to produce soy protein isolates with lower concentrations of isoflavones. In the future, manufacturers may be able to consider processes that modify isoflavone levels from soy protein isolates. Isoflavone levels are not currently labeled on soy infant formula packages.

18. Is bisphenol A (BPA) in baby bottles harmful to my formula-fed baby?

Experimental studies of animals have shown harmful effects of bisphenol A (BPA) on reproduction and development from relatively low-level exposures that may be experienced by infants. Although some studies suggest that BPA exposure can negatively affect brain development and increase the risk for the development of obesity later in life, more research is needed in this area. Recent amendments to food additive regulations no longer authorize the use of BPA in infant feeding bottles and spill-proof cups or the use of BPA-based epoxy resins as coatings in packaging for infant formulas.

19. I remember that many babies in China became sick from contamination of baby formula with a chemical called melamine. Can this happen again, and is internationally produced formula sold in the United States?

In the Chinese incident of contaminated infant formula, melamine was added to falsely increase the apparent protein content because melamine contains nitrogen. This practice has been banned in China. Melamine is not approved in the United States for addition to foods. When the US Food and Drug Administration tested milk (including Yili Pure Milk and Yili Sour Milk produced by Nationwide Hua Xia Food Trade, USA, Flushing, NY), they found melamine contamination. Currently, there are no Chinese-made infant formulas for sale in the United States.

20. How can I limit my baby's exposure to bisphenol A (BPA)?

Avoid clear plastic bottles or containers with the recycling No. 7 and the letters "PC" (indicating "polycarbonate") imprinted on them—many of these contain bisphenol A (BPA). Alternatives include polyethylene or polypropylene that should not contain BPA. Glass is also an alternative but can be hazardous if dropped or broken. Because heat may cause the release of BPA from plastic, it is prudent to consider the following advice:

- Do not boil polycarbonate bottles.

- Do not microwave polycarbonate bottles.

- Do not wash polycarbonate bottles in the dishwasher.

- If pacifiers are used to reduce the risk of sudden infant death syndrome, consistent with American Academy of Pediatrics recommendations, use pacifiers certified by the European Union to be free of BPA and phthalates.

21. Should I stop using canned liquid formula?

The lining of cans may contain bisphenol A (BPA), so avoiding canned formula is one way to reduce exposure. If you are considering switching from liquid to powdered formula, note that the mixing procedures may differ, so pay special attention when preparing formula from powder.

※ If your baby is on a special formula to address a medical condition, you should not switch to another formula because the known risks from the medical condition would outweigh any potential risks posed by BPA. Speak with your pediatrician before you consider changing your baby's formula.

※ The harm associated with giving your baby homemade condensed milk formulas or soy or goat milk are far greater than the potential harmful effects of BPA.

Chapter 3

Safe Drinking Water

It's More Complicated Than Buying a Filter

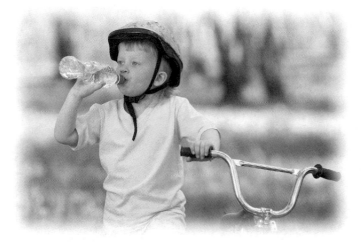

Water Testing, Regulations, and Notices

1. Is it true that federal and state regulations ensure the safety of drinking water?

Federal and state regulations have oversight of water distribution systems that serve at least 25 homes. In most cases, regulations result in very safe water. However, almost 10% of people in the United States drink water that does not meet regulations.

Water safety problems are more common where water supply systems serve fewer than 1,000 people. Some water regulations, such as those for *Cryptosporidium* species, only apply to systems that serve more than 10,000 people.

Information on drinking water quality and violations can be obtained from the water supplier or state health and environmental agencies. Even water that meets all standards may contain harmful contamination. Consumers are given annual written statements of any violations by their public water supply in consumer confidence reports. Many public water suppliers maintain Web sites with current surveillance information. Private wells are not regulated, so determining safety of water from those sources requires the attention of well owners (see Well Water questions later in this chapter).

2. Should I get my water tested?

Under most circumstances, it is not necessary to have drinking water tested. If the local water supply fails to meet a standard, pressure should be exerted on politicians to correct the problem, rather than having people test their own water. Water from wells may require testing (see Well Water questions later in this chapter).

3. **My family's water supply has measurable amounts of some gasoline components that are below the US Environmental Protection Agency (EPA) standard. The community water authority says that the water meets standards and that for further advice, families should contact their pediatrician. What does this mean for my family's health?**

The US EPA sets an enforceable standard or "maximum contaminant level" based on both their best estimate of health risk and the "ability of public water systems to detect and remove contaminants using suitable treatment technologies." Water that meets US EPA standards is deemed to have minimal to no health risk. If you are still concerned, activated charcoal filtration removes benzene and other substances that make up most of gasoline. All filtration systems require care and maintenance.

Contaminants in community water supplies may occasionally exceed standards. If the water is in violation of standards, filtration is a short-term solution, but documenting the effectiveness of the filter is a problem.

A private well that is contaminated with gasoline poses a serious problem because such contamination often represents widespread contamination of groundwater beyond the control of the homeowner. Activated charcoal filtration or a reverse-osmosis filtration may be necessary, but it may be difficult or impossible to make the water safe to drink.

4. **I've heard that nitrate in the water is very bad for us. Are the current maximum contaminant levels strict enough to protect us?**

   Nitrate and nitrite are natural products of the element nitrogen. Nitrate and nitrite are found in some vegetables, cured meats, fish, dairy products, beers, cereals, and drinking water. Most of the population is protected from the harm of nitrate found in water. This harm includes a condition in infants known as methemoglobinemia. The US Environmental Protection Agency's drinking water standards for nitrate (10 parts per million [ppm]) and nitrite (1 ppm) are designed to protect the health even of people who are considered most susceptible. These standards apply, however, only to public water supplies and not to water from private wells.

5. **I've heard of "forever chemicals" that may be in the water, such as perfluorooctane sulfonate (PFOS) and perfluorooctanoic acid (PFOA), that repel oil and water. They may be found in nonstick coatings on cookware and other products. What are the drinking water health advisories that the US Environmental Protection Agency (EPA) recently issued for PFOS and PFOA? If my drinking water has higher levels than those in the advisory, does this mean that my child will become sick?**

   The US EPA reviews scientific studies of laboratory animals and humans and uses techniques to estimate the concentration of a chemical in drinking water that would be safe to consume over a lifetime, called a lifetime health advisory. The intent is for the advisory level to protect against harm in the most sensitive groups, the fetus and the nursing infant.

The current US EPA health advisory for perfluorooctane sulfonate (PFOS), perfluorooctanoic acid (PFOA), or both taken together is 70 parts per trillion (ppt). If a system finds that the drinking water has more than 70 ppt of PFOS or PFOA, then the US EPA advises several actions, including steps to reduce the levels of these chemicals in the water. Drinking water with higher concentrations of these chemicals means that harmful health effects might occur if that water is consumed every day over a lifetime.

6. **Our community had drinking water contaminated with perfluorooctane sulfonate (PFOS) and perfluorooctanoic acid (PFOA) at levels higher than those in the US Environmental Protection Agency health advisory. What kind of medical testing or monitoring should my child have?**

Perfluorooctane sulfonate (PFOS), perfluorooctanoic acid (PFOA), and other persistent perfluoroalkylated and polyfluoroalkylated substances (PFAS) have not consistently been associated with human health effects, despite a large number of scientific studies. Increased total cholesterol level has been found in adults and children with higher PFOS and PFOA levels, but the studies cannot prove causation because many factors that lead to higher cholesterol were not known, such as diet and family history.

No PFAS-specific medical monitoring or tests exist at this time. However, infants and children who regularly go to the doctor have medical surveillance and early intervention for health effects, regardless of exposure to PFOS, PFOA, or other PFAS.

7. I've heard that the health department plans to do biomonitoring in my community because perfluorooctane sulfonate (PFOS) and perfluorooctanoic acid (PFOA) have contaminated our drinking water. What does this mean?

Biomonitoring is used to determine exposure to environmental chemicals, and it involves using blood or urine samples to measure a chemical or its breakdown product(s). A serum perfluorooctane sulfonate (PFOS) or perfluorooctanoic acid (PFOA) measurement is an example of a biomonitoring measurement. Most often, biomonitoring is used in studies or surveys to evaluate which people are exposed to a chemical and to what extent.

For many environmental chemicals, biomonitoring can demonstrate that exposure has occurred, but exposure may not mean that any harm will result. The National Health and Nutrition Examination Survey is an ongoing survey that samples the US general population to evaluate health and nutrition by examining and collecting blood and urine samples from the almost 5,000 participants who are interviewed each year. In addition to clinical laboratory tests, blood and urine samples are used to measure environmental chemicals, including several perfluoroalkylated and polyfluoroalkylated substances (for short, PFAS). Results of these measurements are used to determine reference (normal) ranges (by age-group, sex, and race/ethnicity) to compare with those of individual or group results, to assess effectiveness of actions to reduce exposures, and to track trends in exposure levels in the US population.

8. **I have been notified that the drinking water in my home has perchlorate contamination. Perchlorates, used in rocket fuel, have been found in drinking water and groundwater in many states. I read that high levels of perchlorate can affect the thyroid gland. Should I get my child's thyroid function tested?**

Use bottled water if you have concerns about the presence of perchlorates in your tap water. You may also contact local drinking water authorities and follow their advice. Perchlorate is rapidly cleared from the body, so unless you suspect extremely high levels of exposure, thyroid function testing is likely not warranted.

Babies and Drinking Water

9. **Should I boil my baby's water or use a home water-treatment system?**

If a family uses a public water supply that meets standards, parents should not boil their infant's drinking water or use a home water-treatment system unless the drinking water is contaminated. Drinking water should be boiled only when the water supplier or health or environmental agency issues such instructions. The Centers for Disease Control and Prevention and the US Environmental Protection Agency state that people with special health needs (such as those who have problems with their immune systems) may wish to boil or treat their drinking water. Boiling tap water for 1 minute inactivates or destroys biological agents, but boiling water longer than 1 minute may concentrate contaminants. Point-of-use filters also may be considered but only if they are clearly labeled to remove particles 1 micrometer or less in diameter. Unless they are well maintained on schedule, home water-treatment systems often are ineffective and may even contribute to exposure to waterborne bacteria.

10. How do I know that my water is safe for infant formula?

Water used for mixing infant formula must be from a safe water source, as defined by the state or local health department. If there are concerns or there is uncertainty about the safety of tap water, bottled water or cold tap water that has been brought to a rolling boil for 1 minute (no longer), then cooled to room temperature for no more than 30 minutes, may be used.

11. I have a young baby and will be staying in a vacation home with a well for a few weeks. I do not know whether the well water has been tested. Can I give my baby the well water?

The well water should be tested for coliforms (a certain type of bacteria) and nitrates before being offered to an infant. If this is not possible, it may be safer and more convenient to use bottled water for the baby and others staying in the vacation home.

12. What about testing for lead in water?

If you are using tap water to give directly to an infant or a child, or to make infant formula or juice, or there has been local concern, you may want to have your water tested. To help determine whether your water might contain lead, call the US Environmental Protection Agency's (EPA's) Safe Drinking Water Hotline at 1-800-426-4791 or your local health department to find out about testing your water.

Well water should be tested for lead when the well is new and tested again when a pregnant woman, an infant, or a child or teen younger than 18 years moves into the home. Most water filters, if used correctly, remove lead.

Drinking Water at Home and School: How Do We Know It Is Safe?

13. How do I test my water for lead and what should I do about the results?

Public water systems test for lead but homes may have internal plumbing materials containing lead. Because you cannot see, taste, or smell lead dissolved in water, testing is the only sure way to know whether there are harmful quantities of lead in your drinking water. State or local drinking water authorities maintain lists of laboratories certified for testing drinking water for lead. The US Environmental Protection Agency maintains a Web site providing a list of all such laboratories: www.epa.gov/dwlabcert/contact-information-certification-programs-and-certified-laboratories-drinking-water.

The cost of testing is between $20 and $100. You may also contact your water supplier because the supplier may have useful information, including whether the service connector used in your home or area is made of lead.

A number of steps can be taken to reduce the amount of lead exposure from drinking water at home.

* Use only water from the cold tap for drinking, cooking, and making baby formula. The water from the hot water tap may have higher levels of lead.

- Regularly clean your faucet's screen (also known as an aerator).
- Consider using a water filter certified to remove lead and know when it is time to replace the filter.
- Before drinking, flush your pipes by running your tap, taking a shower, or doing laundry or a load of dishes.

14. Does my pitcher-based water filter remove lead?

Water-filtration pitchers are commonly used because of their affordability. Most water pitchers use granular-activated carbon and resins to bond with and trap contaminants. These filters are effective at improving the taste of water, and many will also reduce levels of lead and other contaminants. Specific contaminants removed vary by model. Carbon filters have a specified shelf life and should be replaced regularly according to the manufacturer's instructions.

15. Lead was found in the drinking water fountain at my daughter's school. Should I have her tested for her blood lead level?

If an elevated water lead level was reported at your child's school, local resources such as the school, health department, or Pediatric Environmental Health Specialty Units (www.pehsu.net) can be contacted to determine if blood lead level testing is needed. It is important to take actions to reduce all sources of lead exposure.

The main source of lead exposure for most US children is from contaminated dust and soil. Schools should work with local, state, and regional resources to establish programs to test for lead in drinking water and other media (such as lead-based paint and soil) and to develop a coordinated health messaging response for families and their communities. The US Environmental Protection Agency has developed a 3Ts (Training, Testing, and Taking Action) toolkit to assist school and child care facilities to address lead in drinking water in their local communities.

16. Is low-grade nitrate contamination a risk for cancer?

We do not know for sure. Published studies of exposure to nitrate in drinking water and cancer risk are not all in agreement, but the International Agency for Research on Cancer has determined that ingesting nitrate in preserved meats (such as bacon, hot dogs, and ham) probably increases the risk for cancer. Although health benefits have been seen with diets that include recommended intake levels of nitrate-rich vegetables, high intake of preserved meats (such as bacon, hot dogs, and ham) is potentially harmful.

17. Do commercial treatment systems sufficiently protect against nitrate contamination?

Water softeners and charcoal filters do not significantly reduce nitrate concentrations. Reverse-osmosis systems and ion exchange resins do remove nitrate but are expensive.

Well Water

18. Should I have my well water tested? How often should I get it tested?

You should test your well water if you have a new baby, have recent damage to the well, or live in a neighborhood where there is known well water nitrate contamination.

As a precaution, people who use private wells that are less than 50 feet (15 meters) deep and who also have septic systems should have their wells tested yearly for coliforms (a certain type of bacteria). In addition to yearly coliform testing, families with private wells should have them tested for nitrates. Risk factors for increased nitrate contamination include shallow well depth, local cropland treated with nitrogen fertilizers, and local animal operations that contribute to regional nitrate contamination.

Collect the sample during wet weather (late spring and early summer), when runoff and excess soil moisture carry contaminants into shallow groundwater sources or through defects in your well. Do not test during dry weather or when the ground is frozen.

19. Our family uses a private well for our drinking water. Should the water be tested for arsenic?

Arsenic occurs naturally in some soil. It also has been used in some pesticides and fertilizers. Arsenic can make its way into drinking water. If your well is a new well, the water should be tested for arsenic and other contaminants. It is recommended that previously tested well water be retested for arsenic every 3 to 5 years, unless there are special circumstances warranting more frequent testing.

20. A leaking underground storage tank at a gasoline station was identified in my neighborhood, and I am concerned that it is contaminating my well water. What should I do?

Strong state and federal regulations developed in recent years require monitoring and abatement of leaking underground storage tanks. A parent should inform the state environmental agency and/or US

Environmental Protection Agency if such a concern is present. Families who may drink water from a gasoline-contaminated source should install activated charcoal filters to their water tap or switch to bottled water. These measures should be taken when there is an unknown source of contamination, when contaminant levels are rising (even though levels still may be below drinking water standards), or when levels of contaminants are steady but higher than drinking water standards.

21. The water from our family well has become contaminated as the result of a spill of "fracking" fluid at a nearby well site. What should we do?

Hydraulic fracturing (or "fracking") involves injecting liquids at high pressures into underground rocks and other structures to extract oil or gas. If there is concern for contamination, it is prudent to use bottled water for all drinking, cooking, and toothbrushing until testing can determine whether your well is contaminated. The state health department should be able to test your water or direct you to where the testing can be done. Call your state health department to discuss whether it is safe to bathe in the water.

Chapter 4

Healthy Eating

From Farm to Kitchen

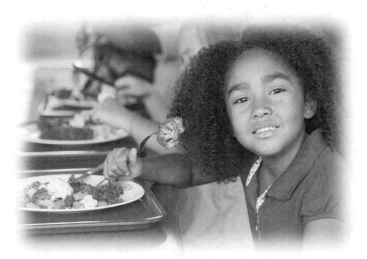

1. **What do the different food labels mean? Are there some that have more meaning than others?**

   Labels of foods have many different meanings and each meaning implies a certain standard of regulation. A good resource to further understand food labeling is "Food Labeling Fact Sheets" found on the US Department of Agriculture Web site: www.fsis.usda.gov/wps/portal/fsis/topics/food-safety-education/get-answers/food-safety-fact-sheets/food-labeling.

2. **How should food be stored or heated?**

   This depends on the type of food. The US Food and Drug Administration has information on safe food handling: www.fda.gov/food/foodborneillnesscontaminants/buystoreservesafefood/ucm255180.htm.

3. **Does artificial coloring cause attention-deficit/hyperactivity disorder (for short, ADHD)?**

   Artificial colors and flavors have not been shown to cause hyperactivity. Research in the 1970s showed a possible correlation between artificial coloring and hyperactivity, but no definitive link was made and more studies are needed. A subgroup of children was shown to have some hyperactivity; this finding has led to current studies to determine why some children are more sensitive.

4. **What can I do to prevent my children from eating products contaminated with prions (the cause of mad cow disease)?**

   Avoid consumption of brains or any food containing nerve tissue. Although no cases of bovine spongiform encephalopathy (mad cow disease) have been reported in the United States, there have been confirmed cases of chronic wasting disease, a brain disease of deer and elk, in western and midwestern states. Avoid feeding children products made with deer or elk from areas known to have chronic wasting disease.

5. **Will food irradiation kill prions?**

No. Food irradiation does not kill prions, the cause of bovine spongiform encephalopathy (mad cow disease).

6. **Are bioengineered food products required to be labeled?**

No. The US Food and Drug Administration (FDA) does not require labeling to indicate whether a food or food ingredient is a bioengineered product. Currently, the US FDA has guidance available for companies that wish to voluntarily label their bioengineered food products.

7. **I know that food irradiation technology uses radiation to improve the safety of food and extend shelf life by reducing or eliminating bacteria, parasites, and insects. Will food irradiation eliminate foodborne illness (usually vomiting and diarrhea)?**

No. Most foodborne illnesses (approximately 67%) are caused by viruses, which are not killed by food irradiation. Among all illnesses spread by spoiled or contaminated food, only about 30% are caused by bacteria and about 3% are caused by parasites. Only about 33% of foodborne illnesses (those attributable to bacteria and parasites) could be prevented by food irradiation.

Antibiotics in Food

8. I know that antibiotics are usually added to the feed given to cows, pigs, and chickens. Do the antibiotics added to animal feed stay in the animals and eventually reach humans who consume meat and poultry?

Antibiotics are often fed to animals to improve growth rates and prevent infections. Many of these antibiotics are also given to people who need them to fight infections. The greater health concern is not that antibiotics in animals remain in food but rather that antibiotics in animals create antibiotic resistance that may be passed to humans. A good example of how antibiotic resistance in animals spreads occurred when pigs developed resistance to the antibiotic colistin. The resistance (via a gene called *mcr-1*) passed to humans in China and was quickly identified in over 30 different countries as well.

To help prevent antibiotic residues appearing in the meat supply, there are regulations requiring specific "washout" periods. Antibiotics must be stopped for a certain number of days or weeks, depending on the drug, before the slaughter of animals or collection of dairy products. These restrictions are designed to prevent animal proteins from containing unsafe residue levels of antibiotics at the time of slaughter or harvest. The success of these regulations depends on the compliance of food animal producers and the adequacy of enforcement and inspection programs.

9. Can animals be successfully raised and brought to slaughter without the use of antibiotics to prevent illness?

Yes. The European Union now restricts marketing of antibiotics for disease prevention in flocks or herds. In addition, some major livestock-producing nations, including Denmark and the Netherlands, specifically prohibit use of any medically important antibiotics to promote growth or prevent disease.

Europe also promotes the use of vaccines, better nutrition and breeding, and improvements to animal husbandry (the science of breeding and caring for farm animals) and hygiene to promote animal health and prevent unnecessary antibiotic use in the first place. In the United States, organic producers certified by the US Department of Agriculture cannot use any antibiotics as a condition of their certification. Use of medically important antibiotics is also prohibited in US poultry production that belongs to the Certified Responsible Antibiotic Use (for short, CRAU) program.

10. Are meat and poultry from animals raised without routine antibiotics very expensive?

Not necessarily. The expense depends on the kind of meat and where it is purchased. In many parts of the United States, parents can buy meat or poultry produced with no antibiotics or reduced antibiotics directly from farmers, at only small price increases from retail supermarket prices. It is possible to identify these producers online or via state and federal programs highlighting community-supported agriculture.

Many school districts with limited food budgets are now buying poultry produced under the Certified Responsible Antibiotic Use (for short, CRAU) label at little to no price increase over other poultry products. The number of fast-food and casual restaurant chains offering chicken products produced with no medically important antibiotics is rapidly increasing. Retail or restaurant products containing pork or beef raised without medically important antibiotics generally are less available or available only at a higher price. Recent announcements by major American meat companies may indicate that the situation is changing in response to consumer demand.

Cooking and Food Storage

11. Can I use glazed ceramic art to store food or beverages?

Glazes may contain metals. Although the lead content of glaze has been limited in dishes made in the United States for commercial sale, some glaze colors used for art projects may contain lead or other metals. These glazes may have labels recommending that they should not be used by children.

Pottery made in some countries, particularly low- or middle-income countries, may contain lead or other metals. Metal contamination has been reported from products made in Mexico and China. Hot foods or acidic foods or drinks stored in such glazed containers may result in leaching of metals found in glaze, resulting in exposure. Glazed ceramic art and pottery from outside the United States should only be used for decoration, not for holding food or drinks.

12. What should I do with my old nonstick (Teflon) cookware?

You may want to dispose of cracked or chipped nonstick pots or pans. Nonstick cookware with cracks or chips is not a good cooking surface and may allow food to stick to the exposed metal surface. Using stainless-steel and iron cookware helps address this concern, but some cooks may prefer pots and pans with nonstick coatings. If used, these pans should be used at recommended temperatures (not on "high") and never be preheated to high temperatures. Above 500 degrees Fahrenheit (260 degrees Celsius), the coatings may degrade and give off fumes. Do not use tools that will scratch and ruin the nonstick surface. Above all, read the instructions that come with the cookware so you can preserve its finish and use it safely.

13. Should I worry about my pizza box? Or microwave popcorn bag? Or fast-food wrapping paper?

Pizza and popcorn boxes, microwave popcorn bags, and fast-food wrapping paper used to be coated with a perfluorooctanoic acid (for short, PFOA)–containing repellent to prevent food leakage and sticking. In 2016 the US Food and Drug Administration (FDA) prohibited the use of several perfluoroalkylated and polyfluoroalkylated substances (for short, PFAS) that were used as paper and cardboard coatings designed to repel oil and water in food containers such as popcorn bags and pizza boxes, as well as food take-out containers and wrappers. Health concerns and environmental persistence were the most important reasons for the US FDA ruling, but the replacement coatings are varied and have not been well studied.

Pesticides in Food

14. Are there pesticides on fresh vegetables found in the store?

Pesticides are commonly found on fruits and vegetables in the store. Because no labeling is required, parents and other consumers cannot tell which fruits and vegetables contain pesticides. Even organically grown fruits and vegetables are not necessarily free of pesticides. It is a good idea to scrub all fruits and vegetables under running water to remove any particle residues left on the surface. Fruits and vegetables are good for children because they provide vitamins, minerals, and roughage. Because of these health benefits, children should continue to consume a wide variety of fruits and vegetables, particularly those grown in season.

15. Are there pesticides in store-bought baby food?

Processed foods generally contain fewer residues of pesticides than fresh fruits and vegetables, in part because federal standards are stricter for processed foods. Some baby food manufacturers voluntarily make their products free of all pesticide residues, although they do not advertise this. Arsenic, a natural metal-like element found in soil, was used as a pesticide in the past. Arsenic has been found in high concentrations in some infant and toddler cereals and snacks. The US Food and Drug Administration has recommended voluntary limits of arsenic in food. Despite this, it is important to provide infants and toddlers a variety of foods.

16. **Could cancer develop in my child because of exposure to pesticides?**

    Many factors contribute to cancer, including genetics, contact with viruses, diet, and environmental exposures. More research is needed to determine how and why cancers develop during childhood. No causal relationship between exposure to pesticides in food and childhood cancer has been established. A number of pesticides can cause tumors in laboratory animals and are associated with cancer in some farmworkers exposed to very high doses.

17. **Are pesticides in foods 10 times more hazardous for children than adults?**

    Many scientists recognize that children may be more susceptible than adults to the effects of pesticides and other chemicals. To account for this difference, which is really an estimate, standards for pesticides in foods may include a 10-fold margin of safety.

Food and Cancer

18. **I heard that hot dogs can cause brain cancer in children. Should my children avoid hot dogs?**

    Sodium nitrite is used as a food preservative and prevents the growth of *Clostridium botulinum* (the bacteria that causes botulism) in meat products. The International Agency for Research on Cancer (part of the World Health Organization) states that consuming nitrate in preserved meats is likely to increase cancer risk. Children should eat a balanced diet, and an occasional hot dog may be a part of that diet. Young children, however, should not be given hot dogs because of the danger of choking.

19. **I am worried that artificial sweeteners will cause cancer, but I am also worried about my child's weight, so what should I do?**

There are 5 nonnutritive sweeteners that have US Food and Drug Administration approval in the United States. These substances are hundreds of times sweeter than sugar, so only tiny amounts are needed to sweeten foods. No studies have shown a link between use of artificial ("nonnutritive") sweeteners and cancer in humans. A study of rats done in the 1970s showed a link between bladder cancer and use of saccharine; however, the way cancer from saccharine exposure develops in rats may not apply to humans.

A wide range of natural ("nutritive") and nonnutritive sweeteners are available in the food supply that can be blended to keep intakes of nonnutritive sweeteners in children well below acceptable daily intakes and reduce excessive calories or other negative effects of nutritive sweeteners. Drinking water is a good alternative to artificially sweetened drinks.

Arsenic in Food

20. **Do I need to limit my child's seafood consumption because of possible arsenic contamination? Are there ever fish advisories about arsenic like there are for mercury and polychlorinated biphenyls (for short, PCBs)?**

The arsenic in seafood is in a form that has not been associated with toxic effects. Therefore, there is no reason to limit your child's consumption of seafood as a way to avoid arsenic.

21. I am worried about arsenic in food products and juice. Do I need to limit the amount of apple juice or rice cereal that I give to my child?

Elevated concentrations of arsenic have been detected in juices—including grape and apple—and rice products. In 2016 the US Food and Drug Administration proposed an action level of 10 parts per billion (ppb) for inorganic arsenic in juice, identical to the US Environmental Protection Agency's 2001 limit for drinking water, and 100 ppb for infant rice cereal. As a precaution, to avoid problems with arsenic in apple juice or rice cereal, it makes sense to vary the source of children's juice and cereal.

Rice cereal is traditionally given to infants as their first solid food, but other first foods include cereals made from other grains such as oatmeal or barley. In addition to containing less arsenic, these other cereals are less likely to cause constipation. Finely chopped or pureed meat (which has iron) and pureed vegetables may also be used as first foods. In addition, rice milk is not recommended for infants.

22. What other steps can I take to limit my family's exposure to arsenic in foods?

A well-balanced diet contains a variety of grains other than rice, such as wheat, barley, oats, and quinoa. To decrease the amount of arsenic when eating rice, rinse it before cooking and cook the rice in plenty of water, as you would cook pasta. Look for rice syrup on food labels and avoid buying products made with rice syrup.

Lead in Food and Cookware

23. We have imported cookware and use imported spices, cosmetics, and ayurvedic medicines. Is it safe to use them?

Some imported cookware contains lead. As the dishes wear or become chipped or cracked, lead can leach from the dishes into foods. The US Food and Drug Administration (FDA) began regulating lead in cookware made in the United States in the 1980s and further strengthened regulations in the 1990s. Dishes made in the United States before these regulations took effect may contain lead.

Some imported spices such as turmeric, cosmetics such as kohl and sindoor, and ayurvedic medicines (these are medicines based on a system from India used for thousands of years) may be contaminated with lead. Because 80% of the spices used in the United States are imported, it is difficult to monitor all spices for contaminants. Although the US FDA is working with other countries to improve the quality of imported spices, cosmetics, and supplements, it always is wise to consider that these products may be sources of lead. When possible, consider using products made in the United States.

24. Is there still lead in canned food?

Cans with soldered seams can add lead to foods. In the United States, soldered cans have been replaced by seamless aluminum containers, but some imported canned products still have lead-soldered seams.

25. How do I know whether fish or other foods contain polychlorinated biphenyls (PCBs) (cancer-causing compounds that are also endocrine disruptors) or dioxins?

Virtually all food today contains trace amounts of persistent organic pollutants (POPs), including polychlorinated biphenyls (PCBs) and dioxins. Commercial foods are regulated, so they should not have more than minimal amounts. Among unregulated foods, the most common source of high-level exposure to POPs is top predator sport fish such as swordfish. States in which exposures to POPs have been a problem, such as those surrounding the Great Lakes, have published advisories concerning the consumption of noncommercial fish, and these advisories are available from state health departments.

It is important for women to eat fish during pregnancy because the omega-3 fatty acids in fish promote fetal brain development. It is also important that pregnant women eat fish that are low in levels of POPs and in levels of methylmercury. Authoritative guides listing the fish that are safe and unsafe to eat, especially during and before pregnancy, have been published by the Monterey Bay Aquarium and the Natural Resources Defense Council.

Herbs and Supplements

26. Medications have many side effects. Should I worry about giving them to my children?

Medicines have been through extensive testing for safety and efficacy by manufacturers and through US Food and Drug Administration review processes, and through these processes, side effects and how often they occur have been identified and are listed in package inserts. Less is known about side effects associated with children's use of certain herbs and dietary supplements because these products do not need to undergo this level of review before coming to the marketplace.

27. Does my child need extra vitamins or food supplements? Won't they help my child grow, eat, and study better?

A diet that provides enough calories and is balanced in all the major food groups generally provides adequate nutrition for an otherwise healthy growing child. Infants and young children may gain dental benefits from fluoride supplements if they drink only nonfluorinated bottled or well water or live in communities that do not add fluoride to public water sources.

Additional vitamin or dietary supplements may be necessary for children to receive the recommended amounts of vitamin D. American Academy of Pediatrics (AAP) guidelines recommend that breast-fed infants and formula-fed infants who consume less than 34 ounces (1,006 milliliters) per day of vitamin D–fortified formula should receive a vitamin D supplement of 400 International Units (IU) per day. Guidelines from the Institute of Medicine (now known as the National Academy of Medicine) and from the AAP recommend that children 1 year and older (and adolescents) have a total of 600 IU of vitamin D daily from food and supplemental sources. Guidelines for supplementation with iron, zinc, and other essential nutrients should be followed.

28. Doesn't the US Food and Drug Administration (FDA) approve herbs and dietary supplements?

No. Laws passed in 1994 made dietary supplements and ingredients exempt from US FDA premarket approval that applies to drugs and food additives. Manufacturers no longer must prove that an ingredient is safe. The US FDA needs to prove the ingredient is hazardous if it believes there is a risk.

29. Is it OK to give my child chamomile or spearmint tea?

Weak teas made from the leaves and flowers of chamomile or spearmint probably pose a minimal threat of harm, although there is little evidence of benefits on children's health from such teas. Keep in mind that children and adults might experience allergic reactions to any plant-derived products such as mint (*Mentha* species) and chamomile (Compositae family).

30. Is zinc of any value in the treatment of colds?

Zinc is an essential metal for good health, and zinc deficiencies can weaken the immune system. Zinc supplementation was recently found to improve the survival of infants who were smaller than is typical at birth. Its value in the treatment of children's colds has yet to be shown in carefully controlled studies.

31. Are over-the-counter herbs of any value in treating my child's colds?

Many laboratory or animal-based studies of certain herbs, such as *Echinacea* or *Astragalus,* have shown them to have remarkable effects on the immune system. However, such results may not necessarily mean that there is a benefit in the treatment of a sick child.

Investigations of the use of *Echinacea* to treat colds in a randomized controlled trial in children showed no benefit.

It is important to understand that some herbal remedies, such as camphor or eucalyptus oil, may be soothing if inhaled but also can have harmful effects, including seizures or coma.

Chapter 5

Your Home

Keeping It Safe for Your Family

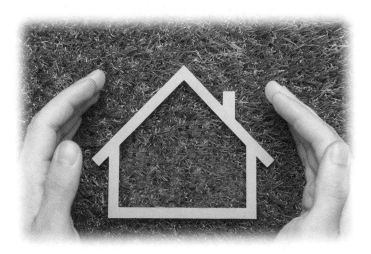

Getting Rid of Pests Safely

1. What is the best way to treat a roach problem?

Hygiene measures are key. Cockroaches are found where there are water and food. Eating should be discouraged in areas other than the kitchen. All food should be stored in closed containers. Water sources should be eliminated by caulking cracks around faucets and pipe fittings. Cracks and crevices where cockroaches can enter the home should be sealed.

A practical approach is to minimize your family's exposure to sprays whenever possible. Individual bait stations are recommended. If possible, baiting should be done outside the home as well. Boric acid, formulated for use as a pesticide, is less toxic than many other chemicals and can be used in cracks and crevices in areas where children are not able to reach.

If these measures are not successful, consult a professional pest control company (exterminator). If professional extermination is to be done, be certain that it is a licensed firm and find out what insecticide will be used and its possible toxic effects. Before using any insecticide in the home, all food, dishes, cooking utensils, children's toys, and clothing should be removed or protected from contamination. After application of the insecticide, young children and pregnant women should stay out of the area for as long as possible. The room should be aired well by opening windows for 4 to 8 hours before people and pets return. Crawling babies should not be allowed in the area until it has been well vacuumed or mopped and residents can be certain that the pesticide was not applied in an area that the infant can reach. For example, if the pesticide is applied to the wall, a crawling infant could hold onto the wall or wipe his hands and have a significant exposure.

Families should avoid using over-the-counter bug sprays and bug bombs. The *Cockroach Control Manual,* an excellent resource, is available from the University of Nebraska. It includes complete information on the least toxic methods for pest control. It is available for purchase or free to download from the Institute of Agriculture and Natural Resources, University of Nebraska Extension in Lancaster County, at http://lancaster.unl.edu/pest/roachmanual.shtml.

2. **We have rodents in and around our home. How can we safely get rid of them?**

Most pesticides for controlling mice and rats (rodenticides) available for home use today are blood thinners. They kill the rodents by causing internal bleeding. These products also can cause bleeding in children if ingested and, therefore, must be used carefully. Each year, more than 7,000 children are exposed to these products; the extent of that exposure makes blood-thinning baits one of the most common pesticide ingestions by children younger than 6 years. Fortunately, the amounts usually eaten by young children rarely cause serious injury. Poisoning can be avoided by following the product label and using common sense.

In 2008, the US Environmental Protection Agency took further measures aimed at decreasing the number of children ingesting rodenticides. "Consumer sized" products may no longer contain certain blood thinners. Using tamper-resistant bait stations with solid bait reduces children's access to these products, and therefore, sales to consumers are only allowed in this form. Because rodenticides have a long shelf life, the older consumer products may remain in use for some time to come.

If you think a child may have ingested a product containing blood thinners, call a physician or Poison Control Center or the emergency department of the nearest hospital immediately.

In addition to rodenticides, pest management techniques include careful sealing of cracks and crevices, cleaning up brush and debris from outdoor areas where rats may hide, and careful cleaning to leave no food scraps for rodents to eat. Mechanical traps can be effective for controlling a minor rodent problem. These include snap traps or glue traps. The latter

Measures That May Reduce the Danger of Children's Exposure to Rodenticides

1. Place all rodenticides out of the reach of children and pets in tamperproof bait boxes. Outdoors, place bait inside the entrance of a burrow and then collapse the entrance of the burrow over the bait.
2. Securely lock or fasten shut the lids of all bait boxes.
3. Use a solid bait and place it in the baffle-protected, lockable feeding chamber, never in the runway of the box.
4. Always use prevention measures along with pesticides to limit rodent access to food and hiding places. Work with neighbors to secure the neighborhood. If baiting alone is used without prevention measures, the rodent population will rebound each time the baiting stops. Prevention measures include using ratproof garbage cans, storing food in tight containers, keeping food in the refrigerator, and frequently raking up garden waste (including fallen fruit).
5. Modify the outdoor environment by rodent proofing buildings and changing landscaping to eliminate hiding places.
6. Continue to monitor periodically to ensure that rodents are not moving back into the area.

are less likely to cause injuries to small children who might come into contact with the traps.

3. **What is the best way to control fleas on a dog or cat?**

There are a wide variety of flea control products, but the safest approach to flea control is to avoid these flea control products altogether because they contain pesticides. This can be done by bathing the pet with a regular pet shampoo at least every other week and at the same time washing the pet's bedding in hot water with a regular laundry detergent. Vacuuming rugs at least weekly is also very important. If your pet is scratching, then carefully comb its fur with a fine-toothed flea comb to look for "flea dirt" and adult fleas. Flea dirt looks like red-brown particles that appear rusty red if pressed onto paper. It represents the blood-filled feces from the fleas. If regular bathing, vacuuming, laundry, and flea combing are not enough to control fleas, then the best option is an oral agent such as lufenuron (Program or Sentinel). The flea products to avoid include flea collars (which generally contain the chemicals tetrachlorvinphos or propoxur) and permethrin shampoos.

4. **My house is overrun with ants. Should I get an exterminator to spray?**

Spraying for ants is generally ineffective. Ants are relatively easy to control by using the principles of integrated pest management, an approach that uses the least toxic methods of pest control and minimizes the use of chemicals. First, it is important to discover how the ants are getting into the house. Once the entry point is identified, it can be sealed off. If sealing off the entry point is not possible, ant bait can be placed in that location as long as it is out of reach of children. It is also important to discover where the ants are going and to remove all food sources by sealing food items in containers or ziplock bags. The ant trail should be wiped clean with dish soap and water to remove the scent that the ants are following. This set of actions causes the ant problem to completely resolve within a few days. If a professional pest control company is needed, look for one that is certified by Green Shield, which maintains standards for integrated pest management pest control (www.greenshieldcertified.org).

5. **My home has bed bugs. Is it necessary to hire a professional exterminator or can I take care of this myself with bug bombs?**

Bed bugs have made a big comeback in the United States over the past several years. The increase in reports of bed bug infestations appear to be the result of changes in patterns of pesticide use and increased international travel. Over-the-counter sprays and bug bombs are not effective against bed bugs.

Sometimes, out of frustration at the difficulty of eliminating bed bugs, people may be tempted to use outdoor or expired pesticides to control bed bugs. Using pesticides not in accordance with the label is a violation of the law and potentially hazardous. Calls to the National Pesticide Information Center regarding poisonings as a result of the misuse of pesticides to eradicate bed bugs are increasing. At least one death has been associated with this misuse. To eradicate bed bugs, consultation with a pest control professional is recommended, as well as practicing integrated pest management techniques.

In the case of bed bugs, integrated pest management strategies include removing clutter, vacuuming furniture and other items that have bed bugs on them, and promptly disposing of the vacuum cleaner bag outside after placing it in a sealed plastic bag. Bed bugs are sensitive to heat. Infested items (clothing, shoes, bedding, blankets, etc) can be placed in a clothes dryer for at least 20 minutes to kill bed bugs and their eggs. Infested mattresses and box springs should be encased in a bed bug–proof zipped cover for 1 to 2 years because bed bugs can survive 18 months without a blood meal.

Arts and Crafts Are Safe, Aren't They?

6. Are water-based art supplies always safe?

In general, water-based supplies are preferable because they do not contain chemical solvents. Unintentionally eating even small amounts of these solvents can be fatal.

Coloring agents used in paints and inks can contain toxic substances such as metals. Some water-based, cold-water dyes are chemicals that cause some people to develop allergic reactions after repeated exposures. Long-term health effects have not been thoroughly studied, and therefore, safer alternatives are preferred. Because some water-based paints may contain formaldehyde preservative, choose formaldehyde-free products. Water-based, unscented markers are preferable over permanent or dry-erase markers. Handwashing is best after using any art product. Make sure to avoid ingestion (such as licking paintbrushes).

7. **I heard on the news that some crayons may contain asbestos fibers. How can I make sure the crayons I buy do not have asbestos?**

The Environmental Working Group (EWG) released a report in 2015 revealing that 4 crayon brands tested in independent laboratories contained detectable levels of asbestos fibers. All 4 crayon types were made in China. The source of the asbestos contamination is from the use of talc, which is used as a binding agent in crayons. The risk of significant exposure to asbestos fibers from the usual use of these crayons is low. When purchasing crayons, ensure that the label does not show talc in the ingredients, the label contains a statement that the product complies with ASTM D4236 (a label created by the American Society for Testing and Materials [ASTM]), and the label has the seal of The Art and Creative Materials Institute. The EWG report was the third study in 15 years to document the presence of asbestos in children's products and highlights the ongoing nature of the issue and need for reform on a federal level. You can view the EWG report: www.asbestosnation.org/facts/tests-find-asbestos-in-kids-crayons-crime-scene-kits.

8. **I am a painter and work out of an art studio in my home. How can I protect my children from potentially harmful exposures from the paint and other materials I use?**

The occupational health and safety of artists, such as painters, is a unique concern because of potential exposures to a variety of toxic chemicals in art supplies and the unregulated setting in which they frequently perform their work (such as the home or studio). Artists may work in small and intensely contaminated home workspaces, leading to exposures for themselves and their families.

Potential hazards in paints and related products include heavy metals (such as lead, mercury, or cadmium), solvents (such as xylene, toluene, or benzene), and others (such as methylene chloride, acids, or alkalis).

Children and family members should be kept out of home art studios and other locations where potentially hazardous materials are used, stored, or thrown away. Home art studios should follow basic principles of hygiene and safety that include selecting less toxic materials when possible, appropriate ventilation, use of proper protective gear, proper cleanup methods, and appropriate storage and disposal of materials. Before reentering other areas of the home, painters should wash their hands thoroughly and change their work clothing and shoes. Details on these principles can be found through agencies such as the Occupational Safety and Health Administration (OSHA) and the US Consumer Product Safety Commission. In addition, OSHA provides free consultations on health and safety practices for small businesses with high-risk exposures (some home studios may qualify): www.osha.gov/dcsp/smallbusiness/consult.html. An organization known as Arts, Crafts & Theatre Safety has a hotline that provides advice about health and safety issues in the arts field: www.artscraftstheatersafety.org/hotlines.html. Some unions, such as United Scenic Artists, provide health and safety information to their members: www.usa829.org/Safety-and-Training/Contact-a-Safety-Rep-for-USA-829.

9. What are safe art materials to purchase for my children?

To ensure that an art material has been evaluated by a toxicologist (an expert in poisons and their effects) for safety, parents should look for materials with the statement "conforms to ASTM [American Society for Testing and Materials] D4236" and has an Approved Product seal from The Art and Creative Materials Institute. Although this label cannot guarantee complete safety of a product, products bearing this label are preferable to products that carry the Cautionary Label. Do not purchase art materials labeled "Keep Out of Reach of Children" or "Not for Use by Children," or that have the words "Poison," "Danger," "Warning," or "Caution," or that contain hazard warnings on the label. Do not use donated or found materials unless they are in the original containers with full labeling. Children should be supervised when using art materials. Materials should be kept properly labeled and stored. Safe cleanup, including handwashing (with soap and water), is important.

Renovating Your Home Safely

10. Our home is being remodeled and the contractor is in the final steps of finishing the project. We recently learned that homes like ours, built before 1978, are likely to contain lead-based paint. What should we do before we move our child back into our home?

Discuss your concern about lead exposure with your renovation contractor. The US Environmental Protection Agency (EPA) requires contractors to be certified in lead-safe work practices to prevent lead dust contamination during renovation, repair, or painting activities in homes, schools, and child care facilities built before 1978. The rule requires the contractor to limit the dispersal of dust during work and leave a clean work site. The contractor must take a dust wipe sample and compare it visually to a reference card. The US EPA "Lead Renovation, Repair and Painting Program" Web page describes the program in detail (www.epa.gov/lead/renovation-repair-and-painting-program).

Individual states may have stricter standards that require surface dust wipe samples to be collected and analyzed in a laboratory. If wipe sample results exceed the US EPA standards of 10 micrograms per square foot (mcg/ft^2) for floors or 100 mcg/ft^2 for interior windowsills, further cleaning is necessary by using a high-efficiency particulate air (for short, HEPA) filter vacuum and by damp wiping all surfaces. When the work site is clean, additional sampling should be performed by a qualified and experienced independent contractor to verify that the cleanup was effective. If the home has a forced-air heating system, it may be necessary to damp wipe the furnace interior and ducts. Carpet, soft furnishings, and ducts with internal duct liners can be difficult to evaluate and decontaminate and may require disposal.

Homeowners with limited financial resources could collect samples for analysis instead of hiring a certified professional; however, lead contamination may be unevenly distributed, so finding low concentrations in one area does not ensure low concentrations in others.

Asbestos also may be present in homes built before 1986 in ceiling tiles, roll vinyl or tile floor coverings, insulation, and other materials. If asbestos-containing materials are disturbed, exposure control procedures are required to prevent asbestos contamination of the home. Contact a local US EPA office for more information.

11. If we install new carpets, can they make us sick?

New carpets may emit volatile organic compounds (chemicals that come off from certain solid or liquids), as do the adhesives and padding that accompany carpet installation. Some people report symptoms including eye, nose, and throat irritation; headaches; skin irritation; shortness of breath or cough; and feeling tired, which may be associated with new carpet installation. Carpet also can act as a "sink" for chemical and biological pollutants including pesticides, dust mites, and molds.

Anyone seeking to purchase new carpet can ask retailers for information to help them select carpet, padding, and adhesives that emit lower amounts of volatile organic compounds. Before new carpet is installed, the retailer should unroll and air out the carpet in a clean, well-ventilated area. Opening doors and windows reduces the level of chemicals released. Ventilation systems should be in proper working order and operated during installation and for 48 to 72 hours after the new carpet is installed.

12. My child has had a persistent runny nose. Could this be caused by the new carpet we installed last month?

A runny nose could be caused by viruses, bacteria, allergies, or perhaps a foreign object in the nose. It also is possible that the symptoms relate to something in the child's environment, such as secondhand smoke or the chemical compounds released from a new carpet. Sometimes an exact diagnosis is difficult to determine. Symptoms from colds are temporary, and symptoms from environmental irritants tend to improve once exposure to the irritant is eliminated. If possible, have your child play and sleep in another room to see if symptoms improve. It may take some time and a visit to your health care professional to determine the cause of the child's symptoms.

13. I saw my toddler eating a piece of lead-containing paint. What should I do?

Bring your child to his doctor's office so they can test him for lead. He may have ingested similar substances even before you noticed him eating the paint chip. Levels of lead in the blood rise rapidly (within hours to days) and can continue to rise as the paint chip moves through the child's digestive system. Once the object has been excreted, the blood level will fall to a new level over the next month. If the child's lead level is 15 micrograms per deciliter of blood or more, the doctor may want to get an X-ray of the abdomen to see if lead is there. If that is the case, the doctor will consult with experts in lead exposure to see about next steps and also will check your child for iron deficiency and treat him with iron if needed.

Depending on how high the lead level is, your local or state health department may become involved to provide education or visit your home to determine the source of lead exposure. It is important to ask about reliable resources in the community to help to resolve the lead problem, if needed; health departments often are not able to provide this service themselves.

Air: What You Need to Know to Breathe Easy

14. What are the most important things I can do to make sure the air in my home is safe for my children?

- Do not smoke and do not allow anyone to smoke in your home. Preventing children from being exposed to secondhand and thirdhand smoke is important. Secondhand smoke is the smoke that others breathe when they are near smokers. Thirdhand smoke is the smoke that stays on clothes or furniture in the home. Do not use electronic cigarettes of similar devices, such as JUUL, in your home for the same reason.

- Keep your home dry and fix all water leaks promptly.

- Woodstoves and fireplaces should be checked yearly by a professional to make sure they are clean and running efficiently.

- A carbon monoxide (for short, CO) detector can be installed on each sleeping level in your home, but this should not be used as a replacement for annual furnace inspections.

- If you have an attached garage, make sure that you turn off the engine and keep the door between the garage and the house tightly closed to reduce the fumes that come into the house after the motor is turned off.

- Gas ovens should not be used to provide supplemental heat because the chemicals they produce can cause breathing problems.

- Children should not come into contact with mothballs because they contain dangerous chemicals.

- Air fresheners do not improve air quality; they use artificial chemicals to provide scent.

15. Are air fresheners hazardous?

Air fresheners release many different chemicals. Some air fresheners contain phthalates, a group of chemicals used in many consumer products. Limited information is available about the potential health effects of using air fresheners. One study linked blood levels of 1,4-dichlorobenzene, a volatile organic compound often used in air fresheners, to lower lung functioning in adults. The long-term effects have not been studied. Scented candles also give off volatile organic compounds.

The list of ingredients may not indicate all the chemicals present in household air fresheners or scented candles. To avoid phthalates, do not purchase products with "fragrance" on the label because these products may contain phthalates.

16. Can plants control indoor air pollution?

Reports in the media and promotions by representatives of the decorative houseplant industry characterize plants as "nature's clean air machine" and claim that research by the National Aeronautics and Space Administration shows that plants remove indoor air pollutants. Although it is true that plants remove carbon dioxide from the air, and the ability of plants to remove certain other pollutants from water is the basis for some pollution control methods, the ability of plants to control indoor air pollution is not well established. The only study of plants used to control indoor air pollutants in an actual building could not determine any benefit. Practically speaking, the ways that plants remove air pollutants seem to be unimportant when compared with common ventilation and air exchange rates. Also, damp planter soil conditions may promote growth of molds.

17. Should I use a humidifier?

Humidifiers should be avoided. A relative humidity of greater than 50% promotes the growth of dust mites and mold. If used, the humidifier must be cleaned frequently to prevent the growth of mold.

18. A compact fluorescent light (CFL) bulb broke on a carpeted floor in our daughter's nursery and we followed the recommended cleanup procedures. Should we have the air tested to determine whether there is a mercury air problem in the nursery?

Compact fluorescent light (CFL) bulbs contain mercury. Air testing following breakage of CFL bulbs is not currently recommended when spill cleanup procedures are followed. Seek additional advice from your local or state health or environmental agency as needed. Following breakage, open windows immediately and carefully follow cleanup procedures (www. atsdr.cdc.gov/mercury/docs/Residential_Hg_Spill_ Cleanup.pdf).

19. What can be done to reduce the levels of particulates from woodstoves and fireplaces?

Exposure to inhaled particles (particulates) in wood smoke may result in irritation and inflammation of the airways resulting in a runny nose, a cough, wheezing, and worsening of asthma. Measures to reduce the levels of particulate matter from a woodstove include ensuring that the stove is placed in a room with adequate ventilation and properly vented directly to the outdoors. Newer stoves are designed to emit less particulate matter into the air. Information on improved woodstoves can be found at www.epa.gov/burnwise.

20. How do I keep my fireplace safe?

There are several suggested measures to increase fireplace safety.

- If possible, keep a window cracked open while the fire is burning.

- Be certain the damper or flue is open before starting a fire. Keeping the damper or flue open until the fire is out will draw smoke out of the house. The damper can be checked by looking up into the chimney with a flashlight.

- Use dry and well-aged wood. Wet or green wood causes more smoke and contributes to soot buildup in the chimney.

- Smaller pieces of wood placed on a grate burn faster and produce less smoke.

- Levels of ash at the base of the fireplace should be kept to 1 inch or less because a thicker layer restricts the air supply to logs and results in more smoke.

- The chimney should be checked each year by a professional. Even if the chimney is not due for cleaning, it is important to check for animal nests or other blockages that could prevent smoke from escaping.

Allergy and Asthma Triggers

21. My daughter has a lot of allergies. Can odors of cooking foods trigger her allergies?

Some proteins released in to the air from foods during cooking may cause reactions in some children. For example, frying an egg or a fish in a pan in a closed area without sufficient ventilation can lead to airway symptoms in children with an egg or fish allergy.

22. Are foam pillows safe for children or can they also trigger allergies or asthma?

All pillows, regardless of content, may serve as reservoirs for dust mites and other allergens. An allergen-proof pillow cover should be used as a physical barrier between dust mites in pillows and the child.

23. My family lives in a multiunit building where there are mice and cigarette smoking in common areas. What can I do about this?

If other families share your concerns about issues such as pest control, mold problems, and cigarette smoking, you may want to organize as a group to alert building management to your concerns for your children's health. Many health departments have regulations regarding problems such as pest infestation and cigarette smoking in multifamily housing, so consult your local health department.

24. I have mold in my home. Should I worry that my daughter is allergic to it?

Testing for sensitivity to mold in children without allergy symptoms is not recommended. Performing these tests in patients who do not have symptoms may lead to an incorrect diagnosis. Positive results of skin tests or blood tests do not necessarily mean that your child has a medical condition. The interpretation of test results must be done in the context of the patient's symptoms. Moldy surfaces should, however, be cleaned, and it is important to fix leaks and other sources of water intrusion to prevent further mold growth.

25. What levels of mold spores in indoor air are acceptable?

There are some rules of thumb for assessing the number of mold spores found in the indoor air. Some investigators have put the average levels of culturable mold counts into 5 groups:

Group 1: Low (<100 colony forming units per square meters [CFUs/m^2])

Group 2: Medium (101–300 CFUs/m^2)

Group 3: High (301–1,000 CFUs/m^2)

Group 4: Very high (1,001–5,000 CFUs/m^2)

Group 5: Extremely high (>5,000 CFUs/m^2)

Air Cleaners

26. Should we use ionizers to clean the air? What about using other ozone-generating air cleaners?

Ion generators act by charging the particles in a room so that they are attracted to walls, floors, tabletops, draperies, or occupants. Brushing up against a surface can result in sending these particles into the air. In some cases, these devices contain a collector to attract the charged particles back to the unit. Although ion generators may remove small particles (such as those in secondhand smoke), they do not remove gases or odors and may not be effective in removing large particles, such as pollen and house dust allergens.

Ozone generators are specifically designed to release ozone to purify the air. Ozone is produced indirectly by ion generators and some electronic air cleaners and produced directly by ozone generators. Although indirect ozone production is concerning, there is even greater concern with the direct and purposeful introduction of ozone into indoor air. No difference exists, despite the claims of some marketers, between ozone in smog outdoors and ozone produced by ozone generators. Under certain conditions, these devices can produce levels of ozone high enough to be harmful to a child. Ozone-generating air cleaners may also contribute to indoor formaldehyde concentrations. They are not recommended for use in homes or schools.

27. Should I consider air cleaners to help clean the air in my home?

Air cleaners include mechanical filters, electronic air cleaners, and hybrid air cleaners using 2 or more techniques. The value of any air cleaner depends on its efficiency, proper selection for the pollutant that is most concerning, proper installation, and appropriate maintenance.

Drawbacks of any air cleaner are that the air cleaner may not remove pollutants completely, may re-disperse the pollutants, may actually mask the pollutant rather than remove it, may generate ozone, and may be noisy. The US Environmental Protection Agency and US Consumer Product Safety Commission have not taken a position either for or against the use of these devices.

The best way to clean air is to remove the source of a pollutant. Air cleaners are not a solution but are an addition to controlling the source of pollutant and providing adequate ventilation.

The state of California regulates air cleaners. The California Air Resources Board lists the models of air cleaners certified by the Air Resources Board as meeting the testing and certification requirements of the state's air cleaner regulation. The certified air cleaner models may be viewed at www.arb.ca.gov/research/indoor/aircleaners/certified.htm.

28. Should I consider buying a portable high-efficiency particulate air (HEPA) purifier?

Some studies have documented that using portable high-efficiency particulate air (HEPA) purifiers can reduce indoor concentrations of particulate matter by about 25% to 50% and reduce asthma symptoms and worsening of asthma.

29. I am about to purchase a new vacuum cleaner for my home. Should I buy one with a high-efficiency particulate air (HEPA) filter?

High-efficiency particulate air (HEPA) filters reduce dust by trapping small particles and not rereleasing them into the air as you vacuum. Vacuums with HEPA filters are widely advertised for use in homes in which children with asthma or allergies are living, but it is not clear whether using a vacuum with a HEPA filter reduces symptoms or medication use of children with asthma. The use of HEPA filters should not substitute for other allergen-reduction methods.

Tobacco Smoke

30. When visitors come to my home, they ask if they can smoke in another room. What should I tell them?

Children's homes and vehicles should be completely smoke-free. Even if smokers smoke in a separate room, smoke-filled air is spread throughout the home and exposes everyone in the house to secondhand smoke. Visitors to your home should honor your request not to smoke during their visit. If they cannot do this, insist that they smoke outside, away from open doors and windows. Thirdhand smoke—the particles that remain on hair, clothing, and skin even after a cigarette is extinguished—is another source of toxicants to your family.

31. I can't stop smoking right now. How can I reduce my child's exposure to secondhand smoke?

Because your child will be exposed to secondhand and thirdhand smoke if you smoke in any part of your home or vehicle, be sure that you only smoke outside the house, and never smoke in your car or any vehicle in which a child rides. Choose a smoke-free child care setting, and avoid taking your child to places where smoking is permitted.

32. We live in my parents' home. They smoke in their bedroom. How can I ask them to smoke outside of their own home?

There are a couple of things you can do. If you feel comfortable (and safe) telling them about how harmful secondhand and thirdhand smoke are to your child, you can say that the pediatrician asked if they would make their entire home smoke-free. Or, if you prefer, your pediatrician can write a note to them asking them to make their entire home a smoke-free zone. Making their home smoke-free may have the added benefits of reducing the number of cigarettes they smoke and encouraging them to take the next step toward quitting.

33. I've tried to quit by using the nicotine gum and the patch before. They didn't work. Why should I try them now?

Nicotine-containing gum and the patch can be used together. The patch controls your baseline urge to smoke. Adding a piece of nicotine gum or a nicotine lozenge in place of a cigarette is used to control any cravings for a cigarette, even if you already are using a patch. Make sure you are using the gum correctly by first chewing it, then "parking" it between the gums and cheek. Some people think that the gum should be chewed like regular gum—but then it will not work. Also, each time you make a quit attempt, you learn more about the quitting process and what works (or does not work) to help you quit. Most people make several attempts at quitting before they succeed. Call 1-800-QUIT-NOW (1-800-784-8669) or your state quit-smoking telephone line and talk with a counselor who will help you plan your next quit attempt. The service is free, and it works.

34. I've heard that the medicine varenicline is very helpful for quitting smoking. What do you know about it?

Varenicline has been effective in helping many smokers quit, but there also are concerns about its safety in some users. It is a good idea to discuss the benefits and risks of using this medication with your doctor or nurse practitioner. Another good source for information is 1-800-QUIT-NOW (1-800-784-8669) or your state's quit-smoking telephone line.

35. We do not smoke but we live in a large apartment building and we smell smoke through the walls. Is this a problem, and if so, what can we do about it?

This is a problem. Children in apartments, on average, have higher levels of nicotine and cotinine, a breakdown product of nicotine, in their bodies than do children in detached houses. Cotinine is a chemical your body makes when you have been exposed to smoke and can be used to measure how much smoke you are exposed to. Potential causes for these higher cotinine levels could be from smoke seeping through walls or shared ventilation systems.

You should consider working for a smoking ban in your apartment building. Smoking bans in multiunit housing may reduce children's exposure to tobacco smoke. A ruling about smoke-free multiunit public housing issued by the US Department of Housing and Urban Development required full compliance with smoking bans in multiunit public housing by 2018. This ruling states that public housing agencies "must design and implement a policy prohibiting the use of prohibited tobacco products in all public housing living units and interior areas (including but not limited to hallways, rental and administrative offices, community centers, day care centers, laundry centers, and similar structures), as well as in outdoor areas within 25 feet of public housing and administrative office buildings (collectively, 'restricted areas') in which public housing is located." Monitoring the implementation of this rule will be important.

36. Are there potential problems with incense burning?

Incense burning in homes can emit particulates, benzene, nitrogen dioxide, and carbon monoxide (for short, CO). Carbon monoxide levels from incense burning can exceed the US Environmental Protection Agency National Ambient Air Quality Standards (standards for outdoor air) depending on the room volume, the ventilation rate, and the amount of incense burned. Incense burning might be a significant contributor to indoor air pollution in cultures in which incense is burned frequently, for example, when people use incense during religious rituals.

A Sea of Chemicals?

37. What do I need to do to my home to prevent my child from being exposed to chemicals that might be toxic?

A child's exposure to chemicals is the sum of what the child eats, drinks, breathes in, and absorbs through the skin. Parents should consider all activities and situations in which a child might be exposed. The home, the child care setting, the school, and other venues may be sources of environmental exposures.

One common environmental exposure is to secondhand tobacco smoke—thus, one of the most important things parents can do is to eliminate their child's exposure to secondhand tobacco smoke. Parents should also know that thirdhand tobacco smoke—the smoke residue remaining on items such as clothing and furniture—may be an irritant. Parents who smoke should be encouraged to quit. Smoking should be prohibited inside the home and smokers should change their clothes and wash their hands before interacting with a child.

The substitutions of environmentally friendly alternatives for household solvents, cleaners, pesticides, and other chemicals are good measures that all families can adopt.

38. What are some other ways to prevent children from being exposed to chemicals?

Prevent unintentional ingestions of toxic materials including those found in some household cleaners. When it is necessary to use such products, store them out of the reach of young children. Products that are not sold in child-resistant containers are likely to be particularly hazardous. Do not store them in other containers, make sure the containers are completely capped during storage, and keep them out of reach. If an unintentional ingestion of a hazardous chemical is suspected, call 9-1-1 and/or immediately take your child to the nearest emergency department for evaluation and possible treatment. For other known or possible ingestions, you also may call the Poison Control Center or (if it is present) the telephone number on the container to receive any instructions on first aid and whether the child needs to be seen at the emergency department for further evaluation and treatment. The Poison Control Center can be reached at 1-800-222-1222.

Whenever possible, avoid products that are more toxic. Household tasks that involve chemicals, including refinishing, paint stripping, painting, automotive work, home hobby work involving lead or solvents, and other tasks that use products that may contain chemicals, should be done when young children are not in the house and by using adequate ventilation before children return to the home (or garage). The California Proposition 65 warning label (https://oehha.ca.gov/proposition-65) indicates products that should be kept out of the reach of young children and that, for the sake of caution, should not be used around them.

Children need safe places to play. Do not allow children to play in industrial sites, either occupied or abandoned. Some of these have been identified as Superfund sites, but even sites not identified as such may have contaminated soil and air.

Be mindful that chemicals in work environments may be brought home on clothing and skin by parents and thus create the potential for hazards to children. When possible, people using chemicals in their work should shower and change their clothes before coming home. When these actions are not possible, avoid contact before showering and changing your clothes and shoes at home, and do not launder work clothes with children's clothing, bedding, and other items.

39. When I bring clothes home from the dry cleaners, are the chemicals released from the clothes dangerous to my child?

Perchloroethylene is the chemical most widely used in dry cleaning. In laboratory studies, it has been shown to cause cancer in animals. Recent studies indicate that people breathe low levels of this chemical both in homes where dry-cleaned goods are stored and as they wear dry-cleaned clothing. Dry cleaners recapture the perchloroethylene during the dry-cleaning process to save money by reusing it, and they remove more of the chemical during the pressing and finishing processes. Some dry cleaners, however, do not remove as much perchloroethylene as possible all the time. Taking steps to minimize your exposure to this chemical is a good idea. If dry-cleaned goods have a strong chemical odor when you pick them up, do not accept them until they have been properly dried. If clothes with a chemical odor are returned to you on subsequent visits, try a different dry cleaner.

Of more concern is whether your home is located directly above or adjacent to a dry-cleaning establishment. If so, the amount of daily exposure may be enough to cause adverse health effects.

40. What are the effects of exposure to mothballs?

Two toxic chemicals, *p*-dichlorobenzene and naphthalene, are used as moth repellents. The active ingredient in mothballs usually is *p*-dichlorobenzene. Exposure to *p*-dichlorobenzene may cause irritation of the eyes, nose, and throat; swelling around the eyes; headache; and a runny nose, which usually subside 24 hours after exposure ends. Reports of prolonged exposure in the workplace to *p*-dichlorobenzene resulted in a loss of appetite, nausea, vomiting, weight loss, and liver damage. Consider replacing mothballs with cedar products, which also repel moths.

41. What is your advice about disposing solvents?

To avoid the problem of disposal, consider using safer alternatives, such as vinegar and water. If you purchase a hazardous material such as a solvent, buy a small amount so that it is more likely that you will use it up completely.

Read the label to find information about the proper storage and disposal of the product. Always follow manufacturer's directions, not only for use but afterward as well. There may be household hazardous product roundups in your community. Many local waste companies offer this service a few times a year. Consider contacting refuse companies found in the phone book or online for more options. Leave the product in its original packaging and seal the container tightly. This will keep the hazardous material from contaminating anything else. Always leave labels intact, even when throwing an empty container away.

Check with neighbors and friends to see whether they have any use for any extra product that you may have, instead of disposing of the unused portion. To prevent unintentional poisoning, keep the product out of the reach of small children.

42. Should I buy an organic mattress for my infant?

An organic mattress should be made with only natural materials that do not contain artificial materials and harmful chemicals such as the flame retardant polybrominated diphenyl ether (PBDE). If you wish to reduce PBDE exposure, several manufacturers now offer mattresses that are free of flame retardants and will decrease childhood exposure to potentially hazardous chemicals.

43. How can I avoid chemicals when I clean my home?

There are numerous sources of information about household chemicals. The US Environmental Protection Agency produced an excellent, user-friendly guide for parents and families that helps with a room-by-room assessment and provides commonsense advice for safer alternatives: www.epa.gov/sites/production/files/2014-06/documents/lesson2_handout.pdf. In addition, the National Library of Medicine has a Household Products Database that is useful: healthdata.gov/dataset/household-products-database.

44. I would like to know how my family can avoid exposures to endocrine-disrupting chemicals (for short, EDCs), such as phthalates and bisphenol A (BPA). What can I do?

There are a few simple steps families can take to reduce exposures to phthalates and bisphenol A (BPA). They include

- Select fresh foods rather than processed foods.
- Look for children's products that are marked free of phthalates and/or BPA.
- Avoid placing plastics in the dishwasher and microwave because high temperatures may promote leaching of plasticizers such as phthalates and BPA.
- Look to recycling labels.
  - No. 3 plastics may contain lead and phthalates. No. 7 plastics may contain BPA.
  - Instead, choose plastics that are labeled No. 1, 2, 4, and 5.
- Choose stainless-steel water bottles rather than plastic. Most stainless-steel bottles have no plastic lining.
- Avoid alternatives that contain chemicals that are similar to BPA (such as bisphenol S or bisphenol F) that also have been found to have endocrine-disrupting properties.
- If using formula, choose powdered rather than prepared canned infant formula.
- Consider using glass baby bottles and glass containers for food storage.
- Dust and mop frequently by using wet techniques, such as a mop or damp rag, to minimize exposure to phthalates in dust.

45. I am concerned about the "forever chemicals," the perfluoroalkylated and polyfluoroalkylated substances (PFAS) that were used in Teflon and many other products to repel water and fat. How can I prevent my child from being exposed to them?

It may not be possible to completely prevent exposure to many perfluoroalkylated and polyfluoroalkylated substances (PFAS) because they do not break down in the environment and can enter house dust, food, and drinking water. Almost all Americans who have been tested have low or "background" levels of several PFAS. However, the use of the persistent PFAS, such as perfluorooctane sulfonate (PFOS), perfluorooctanoic acid (PFOA), and perfluorohexane sulfonate (for short, PFHxS), has declined in the past 30 years and Americans have less exposure now compared with that in the past. It is possible to reduce exposure when there are specific contamination situations involving PFAS. Large drinking water systems monitor for PFOS and PFOA and should notify residents if contamination occurs above specific levels. In this event, residents can use bottled water for drinking. Local and state public health authorities have issued fish advisories, warning people not to consume fish from lakes or rivers that were contaminated with specific PFAS, typically the result of manufacturing runoff or dumping.

46. I am concerned that home dust may be contaminated with polybrominated diphenyl ethers (PBDEs) (flame retardants). Should I get my child's PBDE blood level measured?

Although the level of polybrominated diphenyl ethers (PBDEs) can be measured in blood, the testing requires specialized laboratory staff and complex technology that are not available in clinical laboratories. Because the results do not guide medical therapy or predict future health effects, blood PBDE measurements are not generally available outside of research studies. Routine measurement of blood PBDE levels is not recommended because few laboratories measure PBDE levels, the tests are costly and unlikely to be covered by insurance, and the results do not provide practical information.

47. I just moved to a new house and my neighbors tell me my home used to be a "drug house." How can I find out if the home I moved into was a former secret "meth" laboratory? Could there be chemical residues that can harm my 2 preschoolers?

The Drug Enforcement Administration (DEA) maintains a list of former secret methamphetamine laboratories. It can be accessed at www.dea.gov/clan-lab.

Few studies have shown that exposure to former methamphetamine ("meth") sites results in symptoms that can be attributed to the manufacturing of methamphetamine. If a child has symptoms, a comprehensive pediatric health assessment should be done. Referrals to specialists should be based on symptoms. If the home is on the DEA database, local agencies should be contacted to verify that proper cleanup was completed. If the home is a previously unknown methamphetamine site, environmental testing could be done to assess for contamination.

Personal Care Products

48. What are some online resources that have information about personal care products?

Several Web sites offer information on personal care products, but many have little scientific evidence to support their recommendations. One resource that has been well received by the public and health care professionals is the Environmental Working Group Skin Deep database: www.ewg.org/skindeep. However, errors in interpretation of the science may still occur.

The Cosmetic Ingredient Review allows searching for specific cosmetic ingredients to yield safety information: www.cir-safety.org.

The Chemical Inspection and Regulation Service Web site includes the searchable International Nomenclature for Cosmetic Ingredients list: www.cirs-reach.com/Cosmetic_Inventory/International_Nomenclature_of_Cosmetic_Ingredients_INCI.html.

49. Are plant-based oils safe to use for moisturizing the skin and hair?

Cocoa butter, shea butter, coconut oil, and other plant-based oils are commonly used as hair and body moisturizers. No evidence exists to suggest that these products are unsafe. Like any product, they can cause irritation or allergic reaction in some persons, but if they are well tolerated, they can be a safe alternative to other products that contain multiple ingredients.

The methods used to harvest some of these products, especially palm oil, have raised concerns about harm to the environment. The Roundtable on Sustainable Palm Oil provides certification of sustainably sourced palm oil. Rainforest Alliance certification provides independent verification of environmentally sound practices for harvest of tropical plant products including many plant oils, and Fair Trade certification provides verification of fair labor practices.

50. My 7-year-old daughter is due for her annual physical exam. I have seen news stories about the potential health effects of plasticizers and possible relationship to early puberty. She likes to use nail polish and lotions with fragrance. Given that she already has early signs of puberty, I would like to know what this means for her health.

Generally, puberty is occurring earlier in girls. Specifically, the age at onset of breast budding is occurring earlier, although the age at first menstruation is thought to have remained stable over time. Increasing obesity plays a role in earlier maturation. A variety of endocrine-disrupting chemicals (EDCs) have been shown to either cause delay or promote early development of puberty. Research is ongoing to enhance our understanding of the role of EDCs on growth and development and on puberty because the early onset of puberty is a risk factor for development of breast cancer later in life. Until we know more, it is wise to take a precautionary approach and reduce exposures to EDCs in foods and other products.

51. What about using vapor rub when my baby has a cold?

A few studies have shown that vapor rub use can irritate the airways and increase mucus production. Doctors treated an 18-month-old child in whom severe respiratory distress occurred after vapor rub was applied directly under the nose. Studies of animals whose windpipes were exposed to vapor rub demonstrated that mucus secretion increased and clearance of mucus decreased. Cold symptoms generally resolve on their own and using chemical products, such as vapor rub, will not help resolve symptoms. If you choose to use this product, it should be used according to the directions on the label: only on children older than 2 years and never directly under the nose. Saline (saltwater) nose drops are recommended to help with a baby's nasal congestion.

Specific Hazardous Substances

Asbestos

52. How will I know if there are asbestos materials in my house?

Asbestos is not found as commonly in private homes in the United States as in schools, apartment buildings, and public buildings. Nevertheless, asbestos is present in many homes, especially those built prior to the 1970s.

In homes, asbestos may be found in

- Insulation around pipes, stoves, and furnaces (the most common locations)
- Insulation in walls and ceilings, such as sprayed-on or troweled-on material or vermiculite attic insulation (www.epa.gov/asbestos/pubs/insulation.html)
- Patching and spackling compounds and textured paint
- Roofing shingles and siding

- Older appliances, such as washers and dryers
- Older asbestos-containing floor tiles

To determine whether your home contains asbestos, you can take the following steps:

- Evaluate appliances and other consumer products by examining the label or the invoices to obtain the product name, model number, and year of manufacture. If this information is available, the manufacturer can supply information about asbestos content.

- Evaluate building materials. A professional asbestos manager with qualifications similar to those of managers employed in school districts may be hired. This person can inspect your home to determine whether asbestos is present and give advice on its proper management.

- Test for asbestos. State and local health departments as well as regional US Environmental Protection Agency offices have lists of individuals and laboratories certified to analyze a home for asbestos and test samples for the presence of asbestos.

53. If there is asbestos in my home, what should I do?

If asbestos-containing materials are found in your home, the same options exist for dealing with these materials as in a school. In most cases, asbestos-containing materials in a home are best left alone. If materials such as insulation, tiling, and flooring are in good condition and out of the reach of children, there is no need to worry. However, if materials containing asbestos are deteriorating or if you are planning renovations and the materials will be disturbed, it is best to find out whether the materials contain asbestos before renovations begin and, if necessary, have the materials properly removed. Improper removal of asbestos may cause serious contamination by spreading fibers throughout the area. Any asbestos removal in a home must be performed by properly accredited and certified contractors. A listing of certified contractors in your area may be obtained from state or local health departments or from the regional office of the US Environmental Protection Agency (EPA). Many contractors who advertise themselves as asbestos experts have not been trained properly. Only contractors who have been certified by the US EPA or by a state-approved training school should be hired. The contractor should provide written proof of up-to-date certification.

Children should not be permitted to play in areas where there are crumbling asbestos-containing materials.

To obtain additional information about asbestos in the home, you can read more on the US EPA Web site (www.epa.gov/asbestos/pubs/ashome.html). Information can also be found on the US EPA Hotlines Web site at www.epa.gov/home/epa-hotlines. State or local health departments will have additional information about asbestos.

54. I had my home's air tested and the report shows asbestos fibers. What should I do?

Several different methods of testing for asbestos fibers in air are available and interpretation is complex. Air testing is generally only performed if there is a known asbestos hazard identified from inspection or bulk material testing. Because of the complexity of testing and interpretation, families should consult with one of the Pediatric Environmental Health Specialty Units (www.pehsu.net) or the local department of health.

55. Is there asbestos in hair dryers?

In the past, asbestos was used in some electrical appliances, including hair dryers. However, hair dryers containing asbestos were recalled by the US Consumer Product Safety Commission in 1980, and currently, manufacturers of household appliances in the United States are not allowed to use asbestos.

56. Is there asbestos in talcum powder?

Talc, like asbestos, is a mineral product. Talc from some mines contains asbestos-like fibers, and these fibers are present in talcum powder made from that talc. Because talcum powder is not required to carry a label indicating whether it contains asbestos-like fibers, parents should not use talc-containing products for infant and child care. A further reason to avoid use of talcum powder in the nursery is to prevent talc pneumoconiosis, an inflammation of the lung that can result from unintentional inhalation of the powder if a can were to tip over into a baby's face. Talc pneumoconiosis has been associated with several infant deaths. Women should avoid exposure because genital use of talc has been associated with ovarian cancer and has been classified by the International Agency for Research on Cancer as a possibly cancer-causing product.

57. My spouse works with asbestos. Is there danger to my child?

Any family member who works in an occupation potentially involving contact with asbestos (or similar fibers such as fiberglass or reactive ceramic fibers) may bring home fibers on clothing, shoes, hair, and skin and in the car. These fibers can contaminate the home environment and become a source of exposure to children.

Studies conducted in the homes of asbestos workers have shown that the dust in these homes can be heavily contaminated by asbestos fibers. Mesothelioma, lung cancer, and asbestosis all have been observed in the family members of asbestos workers. In many cases, these diseases occurred years or even decades after the exposure.

Preventing household exposure is essential. People who work with asbestos (such as construction and demolition workers or workers who repair brakes) must shower thoroughly, change clothing, and change shoes before getting into a car and returning home. These procedures are required by the federal Occupational Safety and Health Act but often are not enforced. Workers often are not aware of their exposure. Exposure is prevented only if employees leave contaminated shoes and clothing at the workplace.

Many jobs involve potential occupational exposure to asbestos.

These include

❖ Asbestos mining and milling
❖ Asbestos product manufacture
❖ Construction trades, including sheet metal work, carpentry, plumbing, insulation work, air conditioning, rewiring, cable installation, spackling, drywall work, and demolition work
❖ Shipyard work
❖ Asbestos removal
❖ Firefighting
❖ Custodial and janitorial work
❖ Brake repair

Carbon Monoxide

58. I know that carbon monoxide (CO) is a colorless, odorless, and tasteless gas and that being exposed to CO can result in death. What things can I do to help limit my family's exposure to CO?

Recommendations for Preventing Problems With Carbon Monoxide in the Home and Other Environments

Fuel-burning Appliances

❊ Forced-air furnaces should be checked by a professional once a year or as recommended by the manufacturer. Pilot lights can produce carbon monoxide (CO) and should be kept in good working order.

❊ All fuel-burning appliances (such as gas water heaters, gas stoves, or gas clothes dryers) should be checked professionally once a year or as recommended by the manufacturer.

❊ Gas cooking stove tops and ovens should not be used for supplemental heat.

Fireplaces and Woodstoves

❊ Fireplaces and woodstoves should be checked professionally once a year or as recommended by the manufacturer. Check to ensure the flue is open during operation. Proper use, inspection, and main-tenance or vent-free fireplaces (and space heaters) are recommended.

Space Heaters

❊ Fuel-burning space heaters should be checked professionally once a year or as recommended by the manufacturer.

❊ Space heaters should be properly vented during use, according to the manufacturer's specifications.

continued

Recommendations for Preventing Problems With Carbon Monoxide in the Home and Other Environments (*continued*)

Barbecue Grills/Hibachis

❋ Barbecue grills and hibachis should never be used indoors.

❋ Barbecue grills and hibachis should never be used in poorly ventilated spaces such as garages, campers, and tents.

Automobiles/Other Motor Vehicles

❋ Regular inspection and maintenance of the vehicle exhaust system are recommended. Many states have vehicle inspection programs to ensure this practice.

❋ Never leave an automobile running in the garage or other enclosed space; CO can accumulate even when a garage door is open.

Generators/Other Fuel-Powered Equipment

❋ Follow the manufacturer's recommendations when operating generators and other fuel-powered equipment.

❋ Never operate a generator indoors.

Boats

❋ Be aware that CO poisoning can mimic seasickness.

❋ Schedule regular engine and exhaust system maintenance.

❋ Consider installing a CO detector in the accommodation space on the boat.

❋ Never swim under the back deck or swim platform because CO builds up near exhaust vents.

59. Is using a carbon monoxide (CO) detector a good way to prevent CO poisoning?

Carbon monoxide (CO) detectors are widely available in stores, and consumers may want to consider buying one as a backup but not as a replacement for the proper use and maintenance of fuel-burning appliances (see "Recommendations for Preventing Problems With Carbon Monoxide in the Home and Other Environments" above). The technology of CO detectors is still developing. Several types are on the market, and they are not generally considered to be as reliable as the smoke detectors found in homes today. Some CO detectors have been laboratory tested, and their performance varied. Some performed well, others failed to alarm even at very high CO levels, and still others alarmed at very low levels that do not pose any immediate health risk. With smoke detectors, you can easily confirm the cause of the alarm, but because CO is invisible and odorless, it is more difficult to determine whether an alarm is false or a real emergency.

Organizations such as Consumers Union (publisher of *Consumer Reports*), the American Gas Association, and Underwriters Laboratories have published guidance for consumers. Look for the Underwriters Laboratories certification on any CO detector. Carbon monoxide detectors always have been and still are designed to sound an alarm before potentially life-threatening levels of CO are reached. The Underwriters Laboratories Standard 2034 has strict requirements that the detector and alarm must meet before it can sound. As a result, the possibility of nuisance alarms is decreased. However, you should be aware that some fail to alarm when CO levels are high and some alarm when CO levels are low.

60. What do I do if a carbon monoxide (CO) detector sounds an alarm?

Never ignore a carbon monoxide (CO) detector alarm. If the CO detector goes off,

- Make sure it is a CO detector and not a smoke detector.

- Check to see if any member of the household is experiencing symptoms of poisoning. Symptoms include having a headache, feeling dizzy, feeling sleepy or weak, being short of breath, being confused, or even being unconscious.

- If they are, get them out of the house immediately and call 911. Seek medical attention at an emergency department. Tell the doctor that you suspect CO poisoning.

- If no one is feeling symptoms, ventilate the home with fresh air, turn off all potential sources of CO including oil or gas furnace, gas water heater, gas range, oven, gas dryer, gas or kerosene space heater, and any vehicle or small engine.

- Have a qualified technician inspect the fuel-burning appliances and chimneys to make sure they are operating correctly and that there is nothing blocking the fumes from being vented out of the house. Checking appliances and other possible CO sources should be done before they are turned back on.

61. I recently found out that my furnace has been leaking carbon monoxide (CO), even though I feel fine. Are there any long-term effects?

No data are available that show chronic carbon monoxide (CO) exposure produces any long-term harm. The long-term effects, such as mental and emotional disturbances, only have been described in patients who have had documented evidence of a severe, short-term CO poisoning. Even though you feel fine, it is imperative that you and your family leave the house and have the furnace problem evaluated and fixed immediately. Ignoring this problem could prove fatal to you and your family. If any family members are not feeling well, seek medical attention right away. If you have young children who can't tell you how they feel, it's a good idea to call your pediatrician for guidance.

62. Are carbon monoxide (CO) detectors required in my home?

Many states or municipalities have enacted laws requiring the use of carbon monoxide (CO) detectors in rental units and other residences. The specific requirements vary by state and town.

63. Should I purchase a carbon monoxide (CO) detector for my motor home or other recreational vehicles?

The US Consumer Product Safety Commission notes that carbon monoxide (CO) detectors are available for boats and recreational vehicles and that the Recreational Vehicle Industry Association requires CO detectors in motor homes and in towable recreational vehicles that have a generator or are prepared for a generator.

Lead

64. My child was tested and has an elevated lead level in his blood. How can I eliminate exposure?

In children with elevated blood lead levels, interventions have to be not only effective but also very safe. Work with your pediatrician, who will ask you about potential sources of lead exposure in your home, will test your child for anemia and iron deficiency, and will provide iron supplements if needed. Your pediatrician will talk about making sure your child has the proper nutrition. Your pediatrician will also refer you to your local health department to help identify the lead source and make sure that the source in your home is safely removed. Unsafe renovation practices can further expose children to lead hazards.

65. What are resources for lead?

There are several resources for lead exposure and prevention. Please contact the Pediatric Environmental Health Specialty Units network at www.pehsu.net, Poison Control Center at www.poison.org, or your public health department's childhood lead poisoning prevention program for further information.

66. How can I tell if a toy has lead paint or is made of lead?

Toys are not all routinely tested for lead. Companies that do not always test for lead paint before selling them import many toys from countries with poorly enforced safety rules. The American Academy of Pediatrics advises parents to monitor the US Consumer Product Safety Commission Web site for notices of recalls. Parents should avoid nonbrand toys and toys from discount shops and private vendors. Old and used toys should be examined for damage and clues to where the toy was manufactured. If the toy is damaged or worn or from a country with a history of poor monitoring of manufacturing practices, the safest action is to throw it away. Be particularly attentive to costume jewelry and other small metal pieces that can be swallowed.

Mercury

67. My child swallowed the mercury from an oral thermometer. What do I do?

The mercury in these thermometers is poorly absorbed from the gastrointestinal tract (less than 1% of the amount) and will pass out of the body. No treatment is needed. However, fragments of broken glass are of greater concern for injury. Call your pediatrician right away.

68. Can I throw away compact fluorescent light (for short, CFL) bulbs or regular fluorescent bulbs?

These light bulbs contain a small amount of mercury, much less than a fever thermometer. When they stop working, they should be taken to a hazardous waste recycler or retailer who can recycle them, typically a store that sells light bulbs. Handle the bulbs carefully so they do not break and release the mercury and so you do not get injured from broken glass.

Nickel

69. Should I worry about the nickel in coins, cookware, jewelry, and clothes fasteners? Can my child develop cancer from nickel?

Metallic nickel has not been shown to produce cancer in children. Contact with metallic nickel can cause skin allergies, generally if the metal is in contact with the skin for prolonged periods. Workers in nickel manufacturing plants who inhaled large quantities of nickel salts were found to have a higher risk of cancers of the nose, throat, and lungs. Children are generally not exposed to such high levels from nickel.

Radon

70. Should I test for radon in my home?

The US Environmental Protection Agency recommends that all home floors below the third floor be checked for radon. An inexpensive home-testing kit can be obtained from home improvement stores and from some local or state radon programs. The sample obtained should be sent to a certified laboratory for analysis. Measures to lessen the radon should be taken if the level of radon exceeds 4 picocuries per liter (pCi/L) of air and considered for levels between 2 and 4 pCi/L.

71. What are the health effects from exposure to radon?

There are no immediate medical problems related to radon exposure. However, radon in indoor air is estimated to cause about 21,000 lung cancer deaths in the United States each year. Some studies suggest an increased risk of childhood leukemia with radon exposure. There is no evidence that lung diseases such as asthma are caused by radon exposure.

Chapter 6

Technology

Friend or Foe?

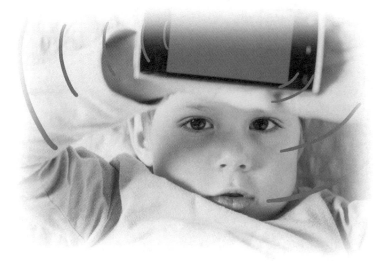

1. **I know that electric and magnetic fields are invisible force lines around power lines, electric appliances, and other electrical equipment. I have heard that electric and magnetic fields may be dangerous. I am about to buy a house, but there is a power line near the home. Should I buy it?**

This is a decision only you can make. Some studies show a link between exposure to electric and magnetic fields and cancer. A cautious approach would include obtaining magnetic field measurements in the home. The measurements sometimes will show that field levels are at approximately the average level despite being near the power line.

2. **I understand science does not have all the answers, but I believe that it is a good idea to avoid magnetic fields when possible. What low- and no-cost measures of avoidance can I take?**

For most people, their highest magnetic field exposures come from using household appliances with motors, transformers, or heaters. The easily avoidable exposures would come from these appliances. If a parent is concerned about electric and magnetic field exposure from appliances, the major sources of exposure could be identified and the parent could limit the child's time near such appliances. Manufacturers have reduced magnetic field exposures from electric blankets (since 1990) and from computers (since the early 1990s). Because magnetic fields decline rapidly with increasing distance, an easy measure is to increase the distance between the child and the appliance.

3. **Is it safe for my children to use a cell phone?**

Experts in some countries have suggested that widespread use of cell phones by children be discouraged.

The American Academy of Pediatrics has recently issued recommendations on reducing exposure among children (see answer to next question).Today's children will have more lifetime exposure than adults to cell phones, so long-term research in this area is needed to fully answer the safety questions. The answer is not fully clear because studies to assess the risk of cell phone use by children, adolescents, and young adults have not been completed.

The levels of energy absorption in children while they are using cell phones is similar to the levels in adults; however, the specific absorption rate of the energy may be higher among children.

Talking on a cell phone during driving or texting during driving results in distraction and increases the risk of automobile crashes with resulting injuries and fatalities. Teenagers and others should not talk on the phone or text while driving.

4. **How can I limit cell phone radiation exposure to myself and my children?**

The American Academy of Pediatrics reminds parents that cell phones are not toys and it is not recommended for infants and toddlers to play with them. Some cell phone safety tips for families are listed below. Additional information can be found at www.healthychildren.org/English/safety-prevention/all-around/Pages/Cell-Phone-Radiation-Childrens-Health.aspx.

- Use text messaging when possible and use cell phones in speaker mode or with the use of hands-free kits.
- When talking on the cell phone, try holding it an inch or more away from the head.

▓ Make only short or essential calls on cell phones.

▓ Avoid carrying the phone against the body like in a pocket, sock, or bra. Cell phone manufacturers cannot guarantee that the amount of radiation you are absorbing will be at a safe level.

▓ Keep an eye on the signal strength—that is, number of bars. The weaker the cell signal, the harder the phone has to work and the more radiation it gives off. It is better to wait to have a stronger signal before using the cell phone. Avoid making calls in cars, elevators, trains, and buses. The cell phone works harder to get a signal through metal, so the power level increases.

▓ If a child plans to watch a movie on the cell phone, download it first, then switch to airplane mode while the child is watching to avoid unnecessary radiation exposure.

5. Do I need to be concerned about exposures from Wi-Fi networks at home and in schools?

Wireless local area networks, or Wi-Fi, use radio waves to connect Wi-Fi–enabled devices to an access point that is connected to the Internet. Most Wi-Fi devices operate at radio frequencies that are similar to those of cell phones, typically 2.4 to 2.5 gigahertz (GHz), although more recently there are Wi-Fi devices that operate at somewhat higher frequencies (5, 5.3, or 5.8 GHz). Radio-frequency radiation exposure from Wi-Fi devices is considerably lower than that from cell phones. The UK Health Protection Agency (now part of Public Health England) conducted a measurement study to assess children's exposures to radio-frequency exposures from Wi-Fi and concluded that exposures were well below recommended maximum levels and there was "no reason why Wi-Fi should not continue to be used in schools and other places."

6. **Is it OK to use white noise from a noise machine to help my new baby sleep?**

Noisy environments can disturb a baby's sleep. Infant sleep machines are designed to provide noises to soothe the baby and to mask louder environmental noises that can interfere with sleep. Infant sleep machines, however, can produce dangerously loud sounds that can harm the baby's hearing, especially if the machine is placed near the baby. If you decide to use a sleep machine, locate it as far away as possible from the baby and never in the crib or on a crib rail, play it at a low volume, and use it for as short a period of time as possible.

Chapter 7

Let's Go Outside!

Playing It Safe in the Yard or on the Beach

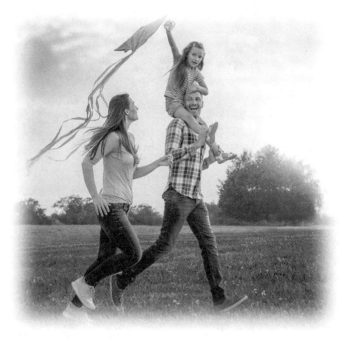

Decks and Wooden Structures

1. **I've heard that wooden decks and play equipment can poison children. Is this true?**

   Chromated copper arsenate (CCA) is a chemical wood preservative containing chromium, copper, and arsenic, used to protect pressure-treated wood from rot caused by insects and by microscopic organisms. Before 2004, many residential outdoor structures, such as playground sets, picnic tables, benches, and decks, were manufactured by using CCA-treated wood. However, because of health concerns related to arsenic, a known cancer-causing substance, the manufacture of CCA-treated products was phased out for residential and consumer uses. Structures currently in use, built with CCA-treated wood before 2004, could potentially be a source of arsenic exposure to children. To reduce exposure, children should immediately wash their hands with mild soap and water after playing on CCA-treated wood.

   Children who touch treated wood or contaminated soils and then touch their mouths or things that go into their mouths may be exposed to arsenic. In several countries that have banned or severely restricted the use of CCA, alternative wood treatments are available. Currently, there is limited availability of lumber treated with CCA in the United States. Coating treated wood with a sealant at least every year (in accordance with wood manufacturers' recommendations) will reduce the amount of arsenic that comes out of the wood. Steps to reduce children's exposure to CCA include

   1. When possible, use alternatives to CCA-treated wood for new outdoor structures, including rot-resistant woods.

2. Keep children and pets out from under deck areas where arsenic may have leached.

3. Do not use CCA-treated wood for raised gardens, and do not grow vegetables near CCA-treated decks.

4. Never burn CCA-treated wood.

5. Make sure that children wash their hands after playing on CCA-treated surfaces, particularly before eating.

6. Cover picnic tables that are made with treated wood with a plastic cover before placing food on the table.

2. What types of sealants or coatings are most effective to reduce leaching of arsenic from chromated copper arsenate (CCA)–treated wood?

Some studies suggest that applying certain penetrating coatings (such as oil-based semitransparent stains) on a regular basis (once per year or every other year, depending on wear and weathering) may reduce the movement of wood preservative chemicals out from chromated copper arsenate (CCA)–treated wood. In selecting a finish, consumers should be aware that, in some cases, film-forming, non-penetrating stains (such as latex semitransparent, latex opaque, or oil-based opaque stains) on outdoor surfaces, such as decks and fences, are not recommended because they are less durable. Talk with someone at a hardware or paint store about appropriate coatings in your area.

Fun in the Sun

Heat

3. Is there a certain temperature at which I should not let my child play outdoors?

Heat indices have been created to identify the health threats arising from the combined influence of temperature and humidity. Air quality indices may be included in deciding whether to avoid outdoor play. These are available at https://airnow.gov and are also typically printed in newspapers and broadcast on television and radio. Along similar lines, cold indices typically combine multiple factors, including outdoor temperature and the windchill factor; these can be obtained from local weather sources. The Centers for Disease Control and Prevention extreme heat guidebook is available at www.cdc.gov/climateandhealth/pubs/extreme-heat-guidebook.pdf.

4. My son has a track meet this weekend and it's going to be very hot. How can I be sure he stays hydrated in the excessive heat?

Recommendations for athletic activities during heat have been published by the American Academy of Pediatrics. During the activity, periodic drinking should be enforced. For children aged 9 to 12 years, 3 to 8 ounces (100–250 milliliters) of fluids every 20 minutes is recommended. For adolescents, 1 to 1.5 quarts (1–1.5 liters) every hour is recommended. Generally, water is good enough to maintain hydration. However, if the exercise is strenuous or lasts for longer than 1 hour, a sports drink should be used.

Sunscreen

5. Why is a baby at special risk from sunburn?

Babies cannot tell you if they are too hot or beginning to burn and cannot get out of the sun without an adult's help. Even dark-skinned babies may be sunburned. Babies need an adult to keep them away from direct sunlight, dress them properly, and apply sunscreen.

6. What can I do to protect my child from the sun?

Babies younger than 6 months should be kept out of direct sunlight to reduce their exposure to damaging ultraviolet (UV) rays. They should be moved under a tree, an umbrella, or a stroller canopy, although on surfaces that reflect light (such as sand), an umbrella or a canopy may reduce UV radiation exposure by only 50%.

To avoid sunburn, infants and children may be dressed in cool, comfortable clothing, such as shirts and pants made of cotton, and should wear hats. Swimwear and other clothing made of materials with high UV protection factor ratings are available for purchase.

Sunscreen should be applied to the parts of the skin that will be exposed to the sun. Parents should apply sunscreen generously and rub it in well before going outdoors, in a way that covers all exposed areas, especially the child's face, nose, ears, feet, and hands and the backs of the child's knees. Sunscreen should be used even on cloudy days because the sun's rays can penetrate through clouds. When choosing a sunscreen, parents should look for the words "broad spectrum" on the label, meaning that the sunscreen will screen out most of the UVB and UVA rays.

A sun protection factor (for short, SPF) of 15 should be enough in most cases. It is important to reapply after sweating or swimming. It is also important to remember that using sunscreen is only one part of a total program of sun protection. Sunscreens should be used to prevent burning and not as a reason to stay in the sun longer. Sunscreen may be applied to infants who are younger than 6 months to small areas of skin uncovered by clothing and hats.

7. I left my bottle of sunscreen in the car for a day. Is it still OK to use?

Temperatures can get extremely hot in a car and may make sunscreen ingredients break down so they are no longer effective. Avoid keeping your sunscreen in a hot car and try to keep the sunscreen bottle covered or in the shade when you are outside.

8. I bought sunscreen with a sun protection factor (SPF) of 30. Does that mean that it is twice as effective as a sunscreen with an SPF of 15?

Although some people believe that a sunscreen with a sun protection factor (SPF) of 30 offers twice as much protection as one with an SPF of 15, this is not the case. When properly applied, SPF 15 sunscreen blocks about 93% of burning rays and SPF 30 blocks about 97%.

More important than SPF is making sure that the sunscreen is labeled as "broad spectrum" and that you use enough (about 1 ounce, or the amount in a shot glass, for an adult or a teen per sitting; use less when applying it to a child, depending on the child's size, but try to use a generous amount). Reapply every 2 hours and also reapply after swimming or sweating. A sunscreen with an SPF of 15 should be enough for most people. Children should wear protective clothing and hats whenever possible and use properly labeled sunglasses to protect their eyes.

9. Can I use a sunscreen spray on my child?

Many sunscreen spray products (like certain other spray products) contain ingredients that can catch on fire, such as alcohol. If you choose to use a spray product, make sure to keep yourself and your child away from any open flame because burns have been reported in people using sunscreen sprays. To avoid inhaling any sunscreen, it is best to spray the product on your hands first, then apply it to the child.

10. Is there special clothing that protects against sunburn?

Some fabrics have an ultraviolet (UV) protection factor rating showing how much sun protection they offer. Even if a fabric does not have a UV protection factor rating, it may offer excellent sun protection. Some fabrics, such as polyester crepe, bleached cotton, and viscose, are quite transparent to UV radiation and should be avoided in the sun. Other fibers, such as unbleached cotton, can absorb UV radiation. High-luster polyesters and even thin, satiny silk can be highly protective because they reflect radiation. A fabric's weave also is important; in general, the tighter the weave or knit, the higher the protection offered. To see how much protection there is, parents can hold the material up to a window or lamp and see how much light gets through. Darker clothes also generally offer more protection. Virtually all garments lose about a third of their sun-protective ability when wet.

11. I am concerned that using sunscreen on my child when she goes outside will lead to a low vitamin D level. Is this true?

Vitamin D helps the body to absorb calcium and so is needed for bone health in infants, children, teens, and adults. The other actions of vitamin D are being studied by researchers. Although vitamin D is made when the skin is exposed to direct sunlight, exposing the skin to the sun's ultraviolet (for short, UV) rays raises the risk for the development of skin cancer.

Fortunately, vitamin D is available from certain foods (such as dairy products, salmon, and sardines) and vitamin supplements. Infants and children should, therefore, be protected from sun exposure with clothing, hats, and sunscreen. To ensure that infants and young children are protected from rickets (a bone disease that occurs when vitamin D levels are very low), the American Academy of Pediatrics (AAP) recommends that all breastfed infants, as well as infants consuming less than 34 ounces (1,000 milliliters) of infant formula per day, receive daily supplementation with 400 international units (IU) of vitamin D. The AAP recommends that children older than age 1 and teenagers receive 600 IU of vitamin D per day. Deliberate sun exposure or using tanning salons as a way to increase vitamin D levels, or for other reasons, raises skin cancer risk and should be avoided.

12. What are nanoparticles in sunscreen?

Nanoparticles are tiny particles used in sunscreen and other products. Nanoparticles in sunscreen are typically zinc oxide or titanium oxide. Titanium oxide in loose powders may be inhaled. If inhaled, titanium oxide has been found to cause cancer in animals. In cream form, it is unclear whether titanium oxide is absorbed through the skin, and there is no evidence that it causes harm. Zinc oxide is not absorbed through the skin.

13. I am concerned about the chemicals in sunscreen and their potential harm to my child. What do you recommend?

Using protective clothing, timing activities, and seeking shade are the most important first-line measures for sun protection. Broad-spectrum sunscreen with a sun protection factor (for short, SPF) of 15 is also recommended. Zinc-based sunscreens (called physical sunscreens) can be a good first choice for parents who are especially concerned about chemical ingredients in sunscreen. Inhaling spray-on sunscreen can be avoided by spraying it into an adult's hand and rubbing it on the child's skin or by choosing sunscreen creams.

Scientific research shows that some sunscreen chemicals are absorbed by people. Studies of laboratory animals show that some chemical sunscreen ingredients have hormone-like effects. Concern has been raised that the vitamin A products retinol and retinyl palmitate, added to many sunscreens, may raise cancer risk. The physical sunscreens titanium dioxide and zinc oxide are increasingly manufactured through nanotechnology, a method that uses tiny particles. It is possible that these particles may be absorbed into the body; there are no studies of children regarding this technology.

These concerns must be weighed against the known risks of sun exposure and sunburning. If you keep these pros and cons in mind, it is reasonable to use sunscreen with the goals of preventing sunburning and possibly decreasing the risk of certain skin

cancers. Sunscreen use should be part of a total program of limiting sun exposure. It may be a good idea
to avoid using products containing oxybenzone, a
chemical with known hormone-like effects, especially
on children.

14. How do I choose sunglasses for my child?

There are no government regulations on the amount
of ultraviolet (UV) radiation that sunglasses must
block. Sunglasses are regulated as medical devices by
the US Food and Drug Administration and may be
labeled as UV protective if they meet certain standards. Parents should look for a label that states that
the lenses block at least 99% of UVA and 99% of
UVB rays.

Protection is provided by a chemical coating applied
to the lenses. Lens color has nothing to do with UV
protection. Ski goggles and contact lenses with UV
protection also are recommended.

It is never too early for a child, even an infant, to
wear sunglasses. Larger lenses, well-fitted and close to
the surface of the eye, provide the best protection.

Playing in the Yard

15. Is there asbestos in play sand?

Play sand that comes from naturally occurring sand
deposits, such as sand dunes or beaches, generally
does not contain asbestos. However, some commercially available play sand is produced by crushing
quarried rock, and this sand has been shown to contain asbestos-like fibers. The US Consumer Product
Safety Commission does not require that the label on
play sand indicate the source of the sand. The label
on sand is not required to carry any information on

whether it contains asbestos-like fibers. For these reasons, do not use play sand unless the source of the sand can be verified or the sand is certified as being free of asbestos.

16. Are the chemicals in swimming pools a health concern?

Concern is emerging about the health effects of chemicals accumulating above a swimming pool, "off-gassed" from the water into the air breathed by swimmers or pool workers. Chemicals, such as chlorine, used in pools are irritating to eyes, skin, and upper and lower airways. Exposure to pool water may also be associated with development of asthma in some children, particularly those with allergies. Children who frequently swim or work in poorly ventilated indoor pools may be at higher risk.

Swimming is a popular and healthy form of exercise for children. Showering before swimming to remove matter such as sweat, dirt, and lotions that can react with pool chemicals to form hazardous chlorine-based chemicals helps to prevent their formation. Proper pool cleaning practices and ventilation will reduce exposure.

17. Should I worry about my young child swimming in a chlorinated pool?

Some studies have shown that repeated exposure to chlorine by-products among recreational swimmers may lead to lung harm. In addition, some studies have been published on the possible harmful effects of swimming on a baby's lung health. Concerns are primarily with indoor chlorinated pools. Long-term studies are needed to clarify this issue.

18. I am having problems with insects in my lawn and garden. Should I get regular preventive applications by a professional service?

Regular lawn treatment exposes people to pesticides unnecessarily. It also may kill insects that help to control the pest population, thereby requiring the use of more chemicals.

Weed killers, especially combination products that include a fertilizer and an herbicide (a chemical that controls or destroys unwanted plants, weeds, or grasses), generally pose an unnecessary risk: they are used for cosmetic purposes but leave a residue on the lawn that can be tracked into the home and may pose a long-term health risk to children.

If a professional lawn service is used, its personnel should (1) regularly monitor the lawn for insects and treat the lawn only when insects are there, (2) offer alternatives to the standard treatment, (3) give advance warning (including to neighbors) before applying any pesticides (this allows time to cover outdoor furniture and remove toys and pet food dishes), (4) be trained and certified, (5) give advance notification of the types of chemicals to be used and information on their health effects, and (6) avoid applications under bad weather conditions (such as high winds).

19. Is an insect repellent containing diethyltoluamide (DEET) safe for children?

Products containing diethyltoluamide (DEET) are the most effective mosquito repellents currently available. DEET also is an effective repellent for a variety of other insect pests, including ticks. DEET should be used in areas where there is concern about illness from insect bites. It also can be used when insects are likely to be a nuisance, such as at barbecues or at the beach. Although it generally is used without any problems, there have been rare reports of harm to children. Usually, these problems have occurred with inappropriate use—for example, if too much DEET is used or if it is not washed off at night; if used appropriately, DEET does not usually present a health risk.

No studies exist in the scientific literature about what concentration of DEET is definitely safe for children. The Centers for Disease Control and Prevention recommends using products with 20% DEET or greater on exposed skin. Use of products with the lowest effective DEET concentrations—that is, between 20% and 30%—seems like the most reasonable choice for infants and young children, on whom it should be applied sparingly. Alternatives to DEET include picaridin (1-methylpropyl 2-[2-hydroxyethyl]-1-piperidinecarboxylate, also known as KBR 3023) and oil of lemon eucalyptus. Picaridin and DEET have similar effectiveness at similar concentrations. Picaridin, derived from the pepper plant, has a favorable safety profile.

The concentration of DEET in products may range from less than 10% to 100%. The effectiveness of DEET plateaus at a concentration of 30%, the maximum concentration currently recommended for infants and children.

The major difference in how well a product works is in how long it will work to keep insects away. Products with concentrations around 10% are effective for periods of approximately 2 hours. As the concentration of DEET increases, the longer it works; for example, a concentration of about 24% provides an average of 5 hours of protection. Concentrations greater than 50% do not provide longer protection.

The safety of DEET does not seem to relate to differences in its concentration. Thus, products with a concentration of 30% appear to be as safe as products with a concentration of 10% when used according to the directions on the product labels. A practical approach would be to select the lowest concentration that works for the amount of time spent outdoors. It is generally agreed that DEET should not be applied more than once a day and should be washed off at the end of the day.

Some properties of infant and toddler skin may differ from those of adult skin until children are at least age 2. Because studies suggest the possibility that young skin may allow chemicals to be absorbed, DEET should be applied sparingly when needed; in addition, the risks of exposure to potentially life-threatening tick-borne or mosquito-borne illnesses should be weighed against the possible risks of DEET absorption. No information is available to show blood levels for infants and children following DEET application.

DEET should not be used in a product that combines the insect repellent with a sunscreen. Sunscreens are often applied many times a day because they can be washed away through swimming and sweating. DEET does not dissolve in water and will last up to 8 hours, depending on its concentration. Repeated application may increase the potential toxic effects of DEET. Sunscreens and insect repellents may be used as individual products applied separately.

Precautions for Using Insect Repellents

1. Read and carefully follow all directions before using the product. Do not allow children to handle the product. When using it on children, apply it to your own hands first and then put it on the child. Do not apply it to children's hands.
2. Wear long sleeves and pants when possible and apply repellent to clothing—a long-sleeved shirt with snug collar and cuffs is best. The shirt should be tucked in at the waist. Socks should be tucked over pants, hiking shoes, or boots.
3. Use just enough repellent to cover exposed skin and/or clothing. Heavy application and saturation generally are unnecessary for effectiveness. Do not use repellents underneath clothing.
4. Do not apply to the eyes or mouth, and apply sparingly around the ears. When using sprays, do not spray directly on the face—spray on the hands first and then apply to the face.
5. Do not apply repellents over cuts, wounds, or irritated skin.
6. Wash treated skin with soap and water when returning indoors. Wash treated clothing.
7. Avoid using sprays in enclosed areas. Do not use repellents near food.
8. If a rash or another apparent allergic reaction develops in a child following use of an insect repellent, stop using the repellent, wash the rash off with mild soap and water, and call a pediatrician or a local Poison Control Center for further guidance.

Chapter 8

What a Beautiful Day in the Neighborhood!

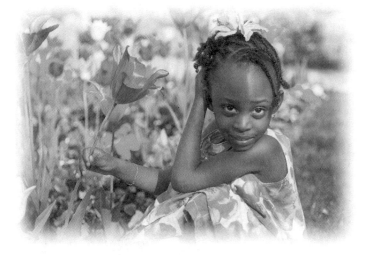

Healthy Neighborhoods

1. We are thinking of moving to a new neighborhood. What can you recommend about what to look for when we are selecting a neighborhood?

Being able to walk or bike to school and other places is good for everyone's health. Consider whether your children will be able to walk or bike to school. Look for the nearest source of fresh fruits and vegetables. Look at the distance to shops and activities and consider whether these locations are close enough for walking or biking. Ask your future neighbors how friendly and connected the neighbors are to each other. Ask whether they see children walking or biking to school. Find the nearest park or playground and consider whether it is within walking distance. Pay attention to the number of trees in the neighborhood.

2. My neighborhood doesn't have a park or any public transportation. What can I do to change this?

In general, to advocate for measures supporting active transportation (such as walking and bicycling), look for helpful community organizations that may include local bicycle coalitions, public transportation organizations, and regional transportation coordination agencies. Local school districts are important partners in advocating for active transportation to school, new school siting, access to green space, and schools' nearness to healthy and unhealthy food outlets. Citizens also can advocate with their city planning departments to make zoning decisions that promote active transportation and access to services such as healthy food outlets, trees and green spaces, and recreational areas.

3. **A drilling company wants to drill for gas immediately next to the playground of my child's school. What should I do?**

Unconventional gas extraction ("fracking") is associated with many health risks. You therefore may want to raise your voice about this proposed well development.

Air Quality

4. **How can I find out about the levels of air pollution in my community?**

Information about the air quality in a community is often found on the Weather page of the local newspaper and is also available through www.airnow.gov.

5. **What can I do to protect my children from the poor air quality in our neighborhood? They want and need to be able to play outdoors.**

The potential harm posed by outdoor air pollution depends on the concentration of pollutants, which can vary from day to day and even during the course of a day. Although exposure to outdoor air pollutants cannot be entirely prevented, it can be reduced by restricting the amount of time that children spend outdoors during periods of poor air quality, especially time spent engaged in strenuous physical activity. For example, ozone levels during the summer tend to be highest in the middle to late afternoon. On days when ozone levels are expected or reported to be high, outdoor activities could be restricted during the afternoon or rescheduled to the morning, particularly for children who have shown sensitivity to high levels of air pollution. In many areas, local radio stations, television news programs, and newspapers regularly provide information about air quality conditions.

6. **Many experts say that we should exercise outside in the early morning to avoid poor air quality that often occurs later in the day. But this conflicts with sports activity schedules. Should organized sports activities be canceled on days when air quality is poor?**

    Children should be encouraged to participate in physical activities because of the many health benefits associated with exercise. In most instances, the health benefits of physical activity likely outweigh the potential harm posed by intermittent or moderate levels of air pollution. However, on hot summer days when temperatures and smog levels are high, this balance could shift, and it may be advisable to shorten or cancel outdoor physical activities, especially for young children.

    When children have asthma, physicians and parents aim for optimal asthma control so that children can participate in normal outdoor sports activities, even on days with poor air quality. When asthma is unstable, children need to limit their physical activities until their asthma becomes controlled again.

7. **My family lives in an area that places them at risk of exposure to increased levels of outdoor air pollution. How can I help my child with asthma?**

    It is very appropriate for you to discuss your concerns about air pollution and other possible asthma triggers with a pediatrician. A child's entire environment, including the home, school, and playground, should be reviewed for possible asthma triggers. Improved medical management of the child's asthma and control of exposure to allergens and irritants in your home may be very effective in preventing asthma exacerbations. If a parent or a pediatrician believes that emissions from a particular facility are harmful to a child with asthma, this information should be shared with the local or state environmental agencies that have authority over operating permits and enforcement actions.

8. Would face dust masks be effective for protecting my children when air pollution levels are high?

Dust masks and other forms of breathing protection, which are sized for adults and not children, are not recommended to protect against outdoor air pollution. Not only do poor fit and uncertain compliance limit any potential benefits, but most simple dust masks do not include the materials needed to filter out harmful chemicals or ozone.

9. I don't understand what is wrong with ozone in the air. Don't we need ozone to block the sun from being too direct?

The ozone in city smog is bad for us, but the ozone in the upper atmosphere is good. Ozone at ground level is a major part of city smog and is hazardous to breathing. The formation of ground-level ozone is independent of ozone in the upper atmosphere (the stratosphere). Stratospheric ozone provides a protective shield absorbing harmful ultraviolet (UV) radiation. We do not breathe stratospheric ozone because it is too high. Too little stratospheric ozone increases the risk of skin cancer and eye damage from UV rays.

10. Are odors from hog farms harmful to children?

Odors mean that chemicals are being released. Chemicals released from hog farms include volatile organic compounds, hydrogen sulfide, ammonia, endotoxins, and dusts. There is good evidence that at high enough concentrations over extended periods, these chemicals can cause disease. Whether the level and duration of exposures from odors released from hog farms are enough to cause harm to children is not known. However, odors can cause increased breathing symptoms and reduced quality of life.

11. If I live in an area with good air quality, is living next to a freeway still a concern? If so, what can I do to reduce my child's overall exposure to traffic pollution?

Levels of traffic pollution are highest during driving on a high traffic road, especially when there is stop-and-go traffic. Even if you live in an area with good air quality, pollution levels can be very high near a busy freeway, and high pollution levels are associated with increased risk of breathing symptoms, including asthma.

A multipronged approach is needed to reduce any child's overall exposures.

- Avoid standing near idling motor vehicles when possible.

- When walking or playing, choose areas away from traffic; even a distance of 300 to 600 feet (100–200 meters) will make a difference.

- Close windows and doors during peak traffic hours and place the air conditioner setting on recirculate.

- Encourage schools to enforce no idling rules at school pickup areas and advocate for switching school bus fleets to non-diesel fuel.

- Support federal and state efforts to reduce motor vehicle emissions. Some state and local governments have adopted laws to limit or require reduction strategies if schools or new residences are built close to busy roads.

12. Is silica the same as asbestos?

No. Silica, or silicon dioxide, is a mineral most commonly called quartz and makes up most of the sand in the world. Breathing in very fine silica particles can cause silicosis, a lung disease that can lead to stiffening of the lungs. Silicosis is almost entirely a disease described in workers without adequate breathing protection who work in mining, sandblasting, or other work that can generate large amounts of silica dust. Children can be at risk if they work as child laborers in such settings. Typical sand on the beach has much larger particles and does not pose a risk of silicosis.

13. We live close to a nuclear power plant. Should I be concerned and take special precautions?

Nuclear power plants are designed and built with public safety as a priority. Emissions from the plant should not require protective actions on your part. However, if you live within 10 miles (16 kilometers) of a nuclear power plant, you may be issued potassium iodide (for short, KI) tablets. In the event of a release of radioiodine, these tablets can prevent radioiodine from concentrating in your thyroid gland. These should be taken only if you are instructed by local emergency management directors. Potassium iodide tablets will protect you only from radioiodine and not from other radioactive substances.

Noise Pollution

14. We live in a neighborhood with a great deal of noise from leaf blowers. What steps can be taken to avoid this noise?

Noise from gas-powered leaf blowers can damage hearing, and exhaust from leaf blowers causes air pollution. Many communities have passed ordinances to ban leaf blowers, but enforcement often is an issue. Work with neighbors and local government officials to educate them about the hazard and create legislation if needed.

15. We live near an airport and the jets fly directly over our house as they take off and land. Will this be harmful to my newborn?

If the noise causes discomfort to you, it may cause harm to the baby. The Federal Aviation Administration maintains a Web site that contains information about aircraft and airport noise and whom to contact with questions, concerns, or complaints about noise issues (www.faa.gov/about/office_org/headquarters_offices/apl/noise_emissions/airport_aircraft_noise_issues). You may also want to seek help from your local government officials. Moving to a quieter setting may be an option for some families.

16. We are thinking of moving to a rural area near a wind farm. I believe in renewable energy but I have heard that wind turbines are noisy. Will there be a problem for me or my family?

Exposure to too much noise can interfere with sleep and cause other problems. Wind turbines generate noise, and a number of symptoms have been described by some people living near wind farms. Exposure to wind turbines seems to increase the risk of sleep disturbances and having feelings of annoyance. The noise decreases as people get farther away from the turbines. Local governments set noise standards for communities. Before you consider moving, it is a good idea to look at where your home is situated in relation to the wind turbines and investigate the regulations in the community.

Landfills

17. My home is near a municipal landfill. Should I be concerned about my child's health?

A municipal landfill usually takes in household waste and nonhazardous material and disposes of them on land. Landfill gases (especially carbon dioxide and methane) can seep out of the landfill and into the surrounding air and soil. These are not harmful to health, but they are considered to be greenhouse gases because they cause global climate change. Many landfills have installed gas collection systems to control these emissions. These gases do not smell, but landfills also release hydrogen sulfide (rotten egg smell) and volatile organic compounds (chemicals that come off from certain solid or liquids). The unpleasant odors from these gases usually keep children away from playing near municipal landfills. It is best to keep your child away from the municipal landfill and to regularly test drinking water from nearby wells.

Hazardous Waste Sites

18. I am confused by the conflicting information I hear about the risks to my children from hazardous waste sites. Can you clarify this?

Hazardous waste sites (sometimes called hazardous waste landfills) are disposal facilities or parts of facilities where hazardous waste is placed. Hazardous waste sites come in many shapes and sizes. Some sites consist of a few abandoned drums, while others may cover many acres. Some are in rural areas and some are in cities. All contain hazardous wastes (wastes with properties that make them dangerous or potentially harmful to human health or the environment). Hazardous wastes can be discarded commercial products, such as cleaning fluids or pesticides, or the by-products of manufacturing processes. In efforts to keep hazardous wastes out of municipal landfills, many communities hold household hazardous waste collection days. You can help prevent hazardous waste by substituting less toxic alternatives in your home, minimizing the use of hazardous chemicals, and advocating for these healthier practices within your local community.

The risks to a child from exposure to a hazardous waste site depend on the amount, type, and length of the child's exposure to the hazardous waste and the types of chemicals involved; because each hazardous waste site is different, the same risk does not apply at each site. It is difficult to know the exact details of a child's exposure, so it is difficult to estimate the risk precisely. For any health effects to be seen, a child would have to have skin contact with contaminated soil, or breathe contaminated air, or drink contaminated water. To prevent health problems, children should not be allowed to play in or near hazardous waste sites.

Explain to children the meaning and importance of posted warning signs, and strongly advise children to stay out of restricted areas. Do not let children swim in streams or other bodies of water that are known to be contaminated. Such conditions usually are posted, but if there is doubt, contact the local health department. Know the source of your household drinking water, and if uncertain about contaminants, have it tested. If you or another caregiver works at a hazardous waste site, soiled work clothes should not be brought into the home. Dust can be a source of exposure for children. Some hazardous waste sites are being cleaned up, and you should stay engaged and vigilant during the development of cleanup plans and the actual cleanup process, to ensure that proper dust control and other safety procedures are in place and followed.

19. Did exposure from a hazardous waste site cause my child's illness? Does that mean that my other child will also become ill?

It is difficult to establish that one child's illness was caused by exposure to one particular hazardous waste site. Most of the illnesses that can be caused by exposure to toxic chemicals have more than one possible cause. A linkage is more likely if several children (or adults) become ill at about the same time, at the same place, and/or following the same exposure.

20. Will my child get cancer from exposure to a hazardous waste site?

Household hazardous waste includes leftover household products that can catch fire, react, or explode under certain circumstances, including paints, cleaners, oils, batteries, and pesticides. Although a number of chemicals found at hazardous waste sites are known or predicted to cause cancer, the chance of getting cancer from exposure to a waste site is thought to be small. If the child was exposed to one or more chemicals that can cause cancer (carcinogens), the risk to the child depends on the amount and length of the exposure and type of carcinogen, among other things. Most experts believe that development of cancer is unlikely unless there has been exposure for many years.

21. Could my child have gotten attention-deficit/ hyperactivity disorder (for short, ADHD) because we live by a hazardous waste site?

A number of chemicals found at hazardous waste sites may affect the nervous system, including a child's developing nervous system. These chemicals include metals (such as lead and mercury), organic solvents (such as toluene), and certain types of pesticides (such as carbamates and organophosphates). The risk to the child depends on how long the child was exposed, the child's age at exposure, the amount of exposure, and the child's genetic susceptibility.

Chapter 9

Oh, the Places They Go!

All Around Town With Your Child

🍃🍃🍃🍃🍃🍃🍃🍃🍃🍃

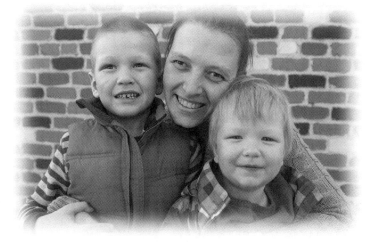

Healthy Child Care

1. **Are there things that the child care center can do to make it safer for my son who has asthma?**

   The 2 most important steps that any child care facility can take to prevent asthma attacks in children are to prohibit smoking and to keep the facility free of molds and other biological pollutants.

   Of the 13 million children 5 years and younger enrolled in child care in the United States, an estimated 1.4 million have asthma (approximately 1 child in 9). Child care programs need specific information on file (provided by the parent or guardian and the child's physician) for every child with asthma. The information should explain known triggers for the child's asthma (such as fragrances, perfumes, pet dander, or pests), medications and how to use them, symptoms indicating when the asthma is worsening, and what to do in an emergency.

2. **The child care center that my baby attends has a sandbox made of wood. Is this safe?**

   Sandboxes are safe if constructed and filled with appropriate materials and properly maintained. Sandbox frames are sometimes made with inexpensive railroad ties, which may cause splinters and may be saturated with creosote, a chemical that can cause cancer. Nontoxic landscaping timbers or non-wood containers are preferred.

   In 1986, concern was first expressed that some types of commercially available play sand contained tremolite, a kind of fiber found in some crushed limestone and crushed marble. There was concern that the long-term effects of exposure to tremolite would be identical to those of asbestos, a cancer-causing fiber. Despite these concerns, the US Consumer Product Safety Commission (CPSC) denied a petition prohibiting marketing of play sand containing significant levels of tremolite. The US CPSC currently has no standards or labeling requirements regarding the source or content of sand.

Directors of facilities may have difficulty determining which sand is safe. They should attempt to buy only natural river sand or beach sand. They should avoid products that are made from crushed limestone, crushed marble, or crushed crystalline silica (quartz) or those that are obviously dusty. When there is doubt, send a sample to a laboratory to determine whether the sand contains tremolite or crystalline silica. Information about reliable laboratories can be obtained from the US Environmental Protection Agency regional asbestos coordinators (www.epa.gov/stationary-sources-air-pollution/asbestos-national-emission-standards-hazardous-air-pollutants#additional-resources).

Once installed, the sandbox should be covered to prevent contamination with animal feces and parasites. Sand should be raked regularly to remove debris and dry it out. A sand rake does a better job than a garden rake.

Chromated copper arsenate (CCA) is a chemical wood preservative containing chromium, copper, and arsenic, used to protect pressure-treated wood from rot due to insects, bacteria, and other microscopic organisms. Prior to 2004, many residential outdoor structures, such as playground sets, picnic tables, benches, and decks, were manufactured by using CCA-treated wood. However, because of health concerns related to arsenic, the manufacture of

CCA-treated products was phased out for residential and consumer uses. Structures currently in use, built with CCA-treated wood prior to 2004, could potentially be a source of arsenic exposure to children. To reduce exposure, children should immediately wash their hands with mild soap and water after playing on CCA-treated wood.

3. **I'm concerned about chemicals in disinfectants that are used in my baby's child care center. What are the best disinfectants for use in child care?**

Although disinfectants and sanitizers are essential to control diseases that can pass from person to person in child care settings, they are potentially hazardous to children, particularly if the products are in concentrated form. Child care standards require a schedule for disinfection practices on items such as diaper changing tables, crib railings, handwashing sinks, and bathrooms (including toilet bowls, toilet seats, training rings, soap dispensers, potty chairs, and door and cabinet handles).

Cleaning products must be stored in their original labeled containers and in places inaccessible to children. Diluted disinfectants and sanitizers in spray bottles must be labeled and stored out of the reach of children. Solutions should not be sprayed when children are nearby so they can avoid breathing in the spray and exposing their skin and eyes.

Household bleach (chlorine as sodium hypochlorite) is active against most germs, including bacterial spores, and can be used as a disinfectant or sanitizer, depending on its concentration. Bleach is available at various strengths. Household or laundry bleach is a solution of 5.25% of sodium hypochlorite. The "ultra" form is only slightly more concentrated and should be diluted and used in the same fashion as ordinary strength household bleach. Higher-strength industrial bleach solutions are not appropriate to use in child care settings. See "Diluting Bleach" table for instructions on diluting bleach with water.

Household bleach is effective, economical, convenient, and available at grocery stores. It can corrode some metal, rubber, and plastic materials. Each state has a water to bleach ratio that is recommended for use in child care facilities. Bleach solutions gradually lose their strength, so fresh solutions must be prepared daily, and stock solutions must be replaced every few months. In child care settings, a bleach solution is typically applied by using spray bottles. Spray bottles should be labeled with the name of the solution and the dilution. Contact time is important. What is typically observed in a child care setting is "spray and wipe." Bleach solution should be left on for at least 2 minutes before being wiped off. It can be allowed to dry because it leaves no residue.

Proper disinfection or sanitizing of a surface requires that the surface be cleaned by (by using mild soap or detergent and a water rinse) before disinfecting or sanitizing. Bleach (the sanitizer/disinfectant) and ammonia (the cleaner) should never be mixed because the mixture produces a poisonous gas. Not all items and surfaces require sanitizing or disinfecting. Guidelines for cleaning, sanitizing, and disinfecting can be found in *Caring for Our Children: National Health and Safety Performance Standards— Guidelines for Early Care and Education Programs* (https://nrckids.org/CFOC).

Diluting Bleach

For use on diaper changing tables, crib railings, handwashing sinks, and bathrooms (including toilet bowls, toilet seats, training rings, soap dispensers, potty chairs, and door and cabinet handles)

DISINFECTING SOLUTIONS

Water	Bleach Strength* 2.75%	Bleach Strength* 5.25%–6.25%	Bleach Strength* 8.25%
1 gallon	⅓ cup plus 1 tablespoon	3 tablespoons	2 tablespoons
1 quart	1½ tablespoons	2¼ teaspoons	1½ teaspoons

SANITIZING SOLUTIONS

For use on eating utensils, food use contact surfaces, mixed use tables, high chair trays, crib frames and mattresses, toys, pacifiers, floors, sleep mats, etc

1 gallon	1 tablespoon	2 teaspoons	1 teaspoon
1 quart	1 teaspoon	½ teaspoon	¼ teaspoon

Disinfection of nonporous, nonfood contact surfaces can be achieved with 600 parts per million (ppm) of chlorine bleach. To make measuring easier, the strengths listed in this table represent approximately 600–800 ppm of bleach for disinfecting and approximately 100 ppm for sanitizing. Chlorine test strips with a measuring range of 0–800 ppm or higher can also be used to determine the strength of the solution. Use a funnel to pour the bleach into the water to avoid air contamination and possible asthma attacks.

Contact your local health jurisdiction for further instructions on cleaning and disinfecting if a specific disease or organisms are identified as causing illness in your program.

*Use only plain unscented bleach** that lists the percentage (%) of strength on the manufacturer's label. Read the label on the bleach bottle to determine the bleach strength, for example, "Sodium Hypochlorite—6.25%" or "Sodium Hypochlorite—8.25%."

Adapted from Disinfecting and sanitizing with bleach: guidelines for mixing bleach solutions for child care and similar environments. https://www.doh.wa.gov/Portals/1/Documents/8340/970-216-Disinfect-en-L.pdf. Washington State Department of Health Web site. Published January 2015. Accessed July 28, 2020.

4. **I'm looking for a child care center near my new home, and the center that is nearest has a smell of cigarettes near the back door. Should I place my child in a child care center if there isn't a "no smoking" and "no vaping" policy in place?**

No. The American Academy of Pediatrics states that in schools, child care programs, and other venues for children, there should be no tobacco use in or around the premises, regardless of whether children are present. Children should not be exposed to vaping or secondhand or thirdhand smoke, and smoke-free policies should be written or stated, enforced, and monitored by the director of the center and parents.

5. **I'm visiting child care centers and I see that many of them have carpets in some of the playrooms. Is this a problem?**

The ideal floor for a child care center is warm to the touch, skidproof, easily cleanable, moisture resistant, and nontoxic, and it does not generate static electricity. This can best be achieved by using hard flooring materials.

Carpets are an easy gathering place for molds and dust mites, as well as lead dust and pesticide residues. Rugs that are secured to avoid slipping on hard surfaces tend to be easier to clean than installed carpeting.

Carpets, pads, and adhesives give off volatile organic compounds (chemicals that come off from certain solid or liquids). For children, especially those with lung conditions, allergies, and allergic-type sensitivities, exposure to fairly low amounts of volatile organic compounds may result in problems such as headaches; nausea; irritation to eyes, nose, and throat; and difficulty breathing.

The child care center should

- Vacuum daily by using a good high-efficiency particulate air (for short, HEPA) filtering vacuum cleaner.

- Leave shoes worn outdoors at the entryway.

- Choose carpet or rugs that clean easily.

- Avoid the use of pesticides on carpeting (some carpeting comes already treated to repel germs).

- Not saturate the carpet when wet cleaning, and ensure the carpet is dry within 24 hours.

- Use low- or no-solvent cleaning products.

- Thoroughly clean and dry water-damaged carpets within 24 hours to reduce molds, or throw the carpets out.

6. **Are air cleaners that generate ozone safe and effective to use in a child care center?**

No. Ozone generators that are sold as air cleaners intentionally produce the gas ozone. Manufacturers and vendors of ozone devices often use terms such as "energized oxygen" or "pure air" to suggest that ozone is a healthy kind of oxygen. It is not. Ozone is a toxic gas. For more information about ozone generators, see the US Environmental Protection Agency publication at www.epa.gov/indoor-air-quality-iaq/ozone-generators-are-sold-air-cleaners.

7. **The director of my child care center often brings in small animals or pets to show the children. Last week, it was a baby goat. Should pets be allowed in child care settings?**

Many child care providers who care for children in their homes have pets, and many centers include pets as part of their educational program. Other than service dogs, animals should be avoided or limited in schools and child care settings.

If a pet is in the child care setting, guidelines to protect health and safety and to avoid risks should be followed. Health and safety concerns for children include allergies, injuries (such as dog and cat bites), and infections (such as *Salmonella* infections caused by common bacteria carried by animals such as chickens, iguanas, and turtles).

8. **I would like to donate my home playground equipment to my children's former child care center. How do I know if it meets regulations?**

Playground equipment is a leading source of childhood injury. Many deaths and injuries have occurred on home playgrounds. Since 1981, the US Consumer Product Safety Commission (CPSC) has worked to strengthen playground safety guidelines and standards. If you are uncertain whether the playground equipment meets US CPSC guidelines, get professional advice. Contact your local parks and recreation office or the National Recreation and Park Association (www.nrpa.org), and they will connect you with a certified playground inspector in the area. This person can determine the safety of the equipment, provide advice about the types of equipment to best suit the ages of the children at the child care center and its physical space, and the type and amount of shock-absorbing surfacing needed around play equipment.

9. **My son's child care center, which has a large play structure built from pressure-treated wood, was recently found to have soil arsenic concentrations of 80 parts per million (ppm). Should I be concerned?**

Cleanup standards for arsenic in soil are established by federal (US Environmental Protection Agency) and state guidelines. State guidelines are highly variable, depending on background concentrations of arsenic in soil, and range from 10 to 1,000 parts per million (ppm). As a conservative measure, lessening or removing the arsenic in the soil should be considered when the soil arsenic concentration exceeds 20 to 40 ppm in areas where children routinely play. Options, depending on concentration, include placement of a ground cover (such as additional soil) or removal. If the source of arsenic is determined to be the structure and not background activity, the child care center also should develop a plan for frequent application of a wood sealant or another barrier while removal plans for the structure are developed.

School

10. **Asbestos was recently discovered in ceilings at my daughter's school. What should the school do? Should we get an X-ray of her chest? What is the likelihood she will get cancer?**

Asbestos was extensively used as insulation in school construction until the 1970s. Because asbestos release is usually episodic—for example, when materials are disturbed during renovation—and usually missed by air sampling, visual inspection is required to establish the nature of the asbestos risk.

All schools must maintain an asbestos management plan and undergo systematic inspection every 3 years. Normally, asbestos removal is not necessary unless children are likely to come into direct contact with it or building renovation is about to occur. More often, the fibers are simply contained by installing drywall, drop ceilings, or other enclosures. Under federal law, you have the right to request a copy of your school's asbestos management plan, which provides information about building inspections, as well as asbestos removal and containment activities. The risk of lung cancer or mesothelioma (a type of lung cancer caused by asbestos) from a brief exposure is very low. A chest X-ray will not be helpful because asbestos does not produce changes in the child's lungs.

11. How do I know if there is a problem with lead in our school?

Schools built before the 1970s are likely to contain leaded materials on walls, woodwork, stairwells, and window casings and windowsills. Other sources include deteriorating paint, lead pipes, lead-lined watercoolers, water fixtures, and lead-containing art supplies. Many children also have potential exposure to lead from drinking water supplied through leaded distribution pipes, present in many cities with long-established municipal water systems. Periodic testing of water at points of intended use can determine the concentration of lead in water. It is reasonable to obtain water for drinking or cooking only from fixtures intended for providing drinking water, instead of from bathroom sinks or utility sinks.

You can contact school officials to ask for copies of any inspections or test results. You also can contact your local health department officials to learn about regulations related to lead hazards.

12. **My kids' school is considering installing artificial turf to save money on maintaining the grass field. They say it is better for the environment. But I'm not sure it is so good for the students. Who is right?**

Today's artificial turf fields are made of the following 3 basic layers:

1. The top layer is a long-pile "carpet" of plastic artificial grass fibers.

2. A second layer of infill material lies within the carpet, to support the "grass" and provide cushioning. It can be made of sand, recycled rubber crumbs ("crumb rubber"), or an alternative material.

3. Underneath is a perforated woven backing holding the carpet in place.

Artificial turf has become a popular alternative to natural grass because of a variety of features.

1. Waste reduction: Scrap tires are a major waste disposal challenge. According to the Rubber Manufacturers Association, in 2007, crumb rubber infill for artificial fields kept 300 million pounds (lb) of tires out of landfills. However, infill must be replaced every 5 to 10 years, so disposal concerns are deferred but not eliminated.

2. Increased hours of playability: Artificial turf fields offer more playable hours than natural grass. Newer natural fields with underlying drainage systems, however, may increase their playable hours and prevent these fields from becoming waterlogged.

3. No need to mow, water, or fertilize: According to a University of California, Berkeley, study in 2010, a 1,000 square foot natural field requires 70,000 gallons of water each week and 15 to 20 lb of fertilizer each year, plus herbicides and pesticides. New natural fields, however, can require less input.

4. Increased access to sports: Artificial fields can be placed on historically contaminated soils to increase access to field spaces.

However, there are health concerns associated with artificial turf.

1. They are hot. Artificial fields are composed of several heat-retaining materials that become much hotter than natural grass. This increases risk of heat-related injuries, such as heat blisters, or illnesses such as heat exhaustion and heat stroke.

2. They contain chemicals. Artificial turf made from recycled tires contains numerous concerning chemicals. These chemicals include but are not limited to chemicals known and suspected to cause cancer (such as benzene, arsenic, cadmium, or polycyclic aromatic hydrocarbons), respiratory irritants, chemicals that harm the nervous system (such as volatile organic compounds, crystalline silica, chromium, particulate matter, lead, or zinc), allergens (latex), and chemicals that harm reproduction (such as phthalates). Children can be exposed through breathing, touching, or eating the chemicals. Exposure is influenced by the age of the field and the environmental conditions, such as temperature, field ventilation, and the child's activity. Chemical composition of fields is highly variable and manufacturers are not required by law to disclose a turf field's chemical content.

To date, limited research shows that these fields do not present dangerous exposure levels. These studies have been small, have not looked into exposure under realistic playing conditions, have not looked into all ways that a child may be exposed, and involve no long-term follow-up of exposed children. Chemical exposures vary according to composition and the age of the field and the environmental conditions, including temperature and ventilation.

Therefore, scientists are not sure about what quantities of these chemicals enter the bodies of active children. Risk may also depend on environmental conditions and field age.

1. Injuries: New fields appear to have similar rates of injury as those of natural grass, although the types of injury may vary.

2. Infections: Artificial turf may have lower concentrations of bacteria but cause more skin scrapes that could lead to infection.

13. Although artificial turf is often composed of partially recycled materials, are there environmental concerns that I should be aware about?

1. Contamination of waterways: Turf fields can leach toxic zinc into waterways, harming the fish and other creatures that live there.

2. Heat island effect: Turf fields may retain even more heat than paved surfaces, worsening the "heat island" effect of cities and communities.

3. Displacement of natural environments: Natural environments offer many physical and psychological benefits. Artificial fields can reduce these natural settings.

Families and communities can research the safest turf options available. They may consult with an expert from the Pediatric Environmental Health Specialty Units (www.pehsu.net) to discuss the newest natural field options. It is prudent to be aware that terms such as "green" and "organic" are not regulated for turf products and have no defined meaning.

14. I understand that the caulk used in some older schools may contain polychlorinated biphenyls (PCBs). What can I do to protect my child?

Until it can be safely removed, limit your child's exposure to caulk containing polychlorinated biphenyls (PCBs) by speaking with school officials about preventing children from touching caulk or surfaces near it. Children should be told to wash their hands with soap and water before eating, and facility janitorial services should use wet cloths to frequently clean surfaces to reduce dust.

15. Someone spilled some mercury at my child's school. How should it be cleaned up?

A specialist should help to clean up even small mercury spills in schools and inside of buildings. Mercury should not be vacuumed or swept up because this may spread the mercury droplets and increase mercury vapor. Keep everyone out of the room where the mercury spilled. Children and pregnant women should not be allowed to help, and windows and doors in the affected rooms should be opened to the outside and closed off from other rooms. If the spilled amount is small, such as from a broken thermometer, it may be cleaned up by using a damp rag or paper towels (www.epa.gov/mercury/what-do-if-mercury-thermometer-breaks). If the amount of mercury appears to be more than 2 table-spoons (30 milliliters), the National Response Center (NRC) should be called for assistance. The NRC hotline operates 24 hours a day, 7 days a week. Call 1-800-424-8802. Your local health department may be able to assist.

16. **I understand that some buildings have high levels of radon, a gas that causes cancer. My home radon test result was elevated, and it made me wonder if the school nearby is tested. Is this a requirement?**

Before the COVID-19 pandemic, children spent a third or more of their weekdays in schools; the length of time they spend there makes radon in schools a potential concern. The US Environmental Protection Agency recommends that all schools be tested for radon. Radon problems in schools are often remedied by adjusting settings of central ventilation systems. More detailed information is available at www.epa.gov/iaq-schools/managing-radon-schools.

17. **I think my child is being made sick by the chemicals that she is exposed to in school. Can my pediatrician intervene and help me talk with the school about chemicals in the school?**

If you are concerned, your child's doctor should perform a thorough history and physical examination of your child as an essential first step.

Your pediatrician can be proactive in working closely with the parents and the school officials toward an assessment of the school environment and an educational solution that serves the best interests of your child. A Pediatric Environmental Health Specialty Unit (www.pehsu.net) and local and/or state health department officials may be of assistance as additional resources.

Around Town

18. What is the risk to my child of exposure to gasoline vapors when she is in the car while I am at a service station filling the tank with gasoline?

The risk is minimal, but exposure should be kept as brief as possible to minimize risk of delayed consequences, especially leukemia caused by breathing in benzene vapor. Closing the windows is recommended. Adults should not hold infants while fueling vehicles. Some states regulate the age at which children can fuel cars, with age limits typically 16 years or older.

19. I took my family to a wedding reception where the music was so loud that I could not hear the person who was sitting at the table next to me. Isn't this level of noise bad for our ears?

Many weddings and similar celebratory events have excessively loud band or DJ music. The music volume at these events often is uncomfortable or causes ear pain. It is helpful in these situations to have earplugs with you (and for family members) or to temporarily relocate while the music is playing. Asking the host to have the band or DJ lower the volume may result in some relief. You are also pointing out a larger issue: if noise was more widely understood as a major public health problem, then situations such as this would be less likely to arise. Unfortunately, many people appear to relish being in an extremely noisy music environment. A long-term approach of education and regulation is needed to avoid these situations in the future.

Chapter 10

Your Teenager

A Whole New World

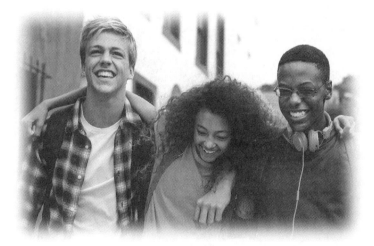

1. **My teenager seems to constantly be using
    either earbuds or headphones. Will this harm
    her hearing?**

    There are several reports of hearing loss after the use
    of personal audio players using either headphones
    or earbuds. Children and adolescents should be
    educated about the potential danger of loud music,
    whether heard at concerts, dances, and other social
    events or through earbuds or headphones. The
    personal digital audio player should be set at approx-
    imately 60% of maximum volume (maximum volume
    is about 100–110 decibels, a measure of the noise
    level), and listening should be limited to 60 minutes
    daily. The user should be able to hear conversations
    going on around him or her while listening to the
    music. Earbuds generally have tighter seals with the
    ear canal than do headphones, so sound transfer may
    be more efficient with earbuds. Ringing or a feeling
    of fullness in the ear definitely means the music was
    too loud.

2. **A rash developed on my teen's hands and back.
    I found him sleeping on his iPad, and I wonder if
    he has an allergy to metal in his iPad.**

    Allergic contact dermatitis (a rash resulting from
    skin contact with something a person is allergic to)
    has been known to occur from the use of handheld
    devices. This is usually caused by a nickel allergy, but
    contact with other metals may result in a rash. Nickel
    allergy is becoming more common in the United
    States, so parents should be aware of the presence
    of this metal in these devices. Nickel-free cases are
    available. Using a cover regularly in this situation
    is recommended.

3. Is using a spray tan safe?

"Spray tans," also known as "sunless" or "self-tanning" products, are sometimes used by people to substitute for going outside or visiting a tanning salon. Sunless tanners use dihydroxyacetone (DHA), a chemical that reacts to the top layer of skin to form brown-black compounds (melanoidins) that deposit in the skin. Dihydroxyacetone is a chemical that induces DNA strand breaks in certain strains of bacteria; it has not been shown to cause cancer in animals. Dihydroxyacetone is the only color additive approved by the US Food and Drug Administration for use as a tanning agent. Dihydroxyacetone–containing tanning preparations may be applied to the consumer's bare skin by misters at sunless tanning booths. Bronzers are water-soluble dyes that temporarily stain the skin. Bronzers are easily removed with soap and water.

Dihydroxyacetone–induced tans become apparent within 1 hour; maximal darkening occurs within 8 to 24 hours. Most users report that color disappears over 5 to 7 days. Neither DHA nor melanoidins provide any significant protection from the ultraviolet (UV) radiation coming from the sun. Therefore, consumers must be advised that sunburn and sun damage may occur unless they use sunscreen and other sun protection methods when they are outdoors. Consumers must also be warned that any sunless products containing added sunscreen only provide UV radiation protection during a few hours after application and that additional sun protection must be used during the duration of the artificial tan. Potential spray tan users may also be advised that it is probably healthier to "love the skin you're in" rather than seeking a darker look.

4. Are tanning salons safe?

People who use sunlamps or go to tanning salons are exposed primarily to ultraviolet (UV) A radiation that comes from the tanning lamps. The tan that occurs represents a protective response to the harmful UV rays. Skin damage occurs whether a tan comes from the sun itself or from artificial light from a tanning salon. Tanning in a tanning salon (or other places such as gyms) raises the risk for the development of skin cancer. Tanning salons are not safe and should not be used by teenagers or others. The American Academy of Pediatrics, the World Health Organization, the American Academy of Dermatology, and the American Medical Association have urged states to pass legislation that prohibits minors younger than 18 years from accessing tanning salons.

5. I've heard that vaping products are safer for teens to use than regular cigarettes. Is this true?

This is not true. Scientific studies are showing that teens who previously never smoked are more likely to use regular cigarettes after they start using electronic cigarettes. Teens' brains are still developing, so they are prone to become addicted to the nicotine contained in electronic cigarettes and similar electronic devices that deliver nicotine. They then often go on to use traditional cigarettes and become addicted to them. Using electronic cigarettes is hazardous for teens and is not recommended. Vaping has also been linked to serious lung injury.

6. Are electronic cigarettes effective for stopping smoking?

The research to date suggests that among adults who want to stop smoking, electronic cigarettes provide minimal if any benefit. Studies suggest that smokers who use electronic cigarettes are less likely to stop smoking than those individuals who do not use electronic cigarettes. Among adolescents, use of electronic cigarettes increases the progression of tobacco dependence and decreases the likelihood of stopping smoking.

7. Is hookah smoking less harmful than cigarette smoking? Does bubbling the smoke through water remove the toxicants?

Hookah smoking is as harmful—if not more harmful—than cigarette smoking. Passing the smoke through water does not remove the toxic chemicals and the chemicals that cause cancer. The charcoal used to heat the tobacco can raise health risks by producing high levels of carbon monoxide (for short, CO), metals, and cancer-causing chemicals.

Because of the way a hookah is used, smokers may absorb more of the toxic substances also found in cigarette smoke than cigarette smokers do. An hour-long hookah smoking session involves 200 puffs, whereas smoking an average cigarette involves 20 puffs. The amount of smoke inhaled during a typical hookah session is about 90,000 milliliters (mL), compared with 500 to 600 mL inhaled during smoking a cigarette.

8. **Are there risks to electronic cigarettes that use a solution that does not contain nicotine?**

Inaccurate labeling on these products has been identified. Electronic cigarette products marketed as being nicotine-free have been found to contain nicotine. Electronic cigarette products deliver other toxic chemicals in their emissions, including metallic nanoparticles, chemicals that cause cancer, and volatile organic compounds. Many of the flavoring agents used are breathing irritants and can be damaging to respiratory lung tissues when inhaled. With or without nicotine, the emissions from electronic cigarette devices are not safe to inhale.

9. **What are the long-term risks of gasoline sniffing to children and adolescents?**

Mental deterioration and permanent injury to the nervous system are the principal health dangers of chronic abuse of solvents, including gasoline. This leads to trouble with attention, memory, and problem-solving, as well as muscle weakness, tremor, and balance problems. The mood of the person changes as dementia develops. There are effects on the kidney. Chronic gasoline sniffing also causes certain cancers. Gasoline sniffing is a marker that a child or teenager is at very high risk of trying or already using other drugs.

10. **My teenager has asthma, for which she takes daily medication. She wants to get a part-time job. Can I help direct her to work that won't cause her asthma to flare up?**

Teenagers need to ask potential employers about the tasks they will be doing and whether they may be exposed to any chemical lung irritants, cold, or allergens. Although increasingly infrequent because of indoor smoking bans in many states, a restaurant with a smoking section is not a wise choice for a teenager with asthma. A customer service or cashier job should provide a better breathing environment, or the teenager with asthma may seek work in an ice cream store that does not allow smoking, as long as the use of cleaning materials that are lung irritants is not also required. In any job, parents should be concerned about adult supervision, job training, and safety training. It is important for parents to visit the workplace. A job that requires personal protective equipment suggests a possible risk that should be explored and discussed with the adolescent. Potential chemical exposures in vocational education, shop or art classes, work-study programs, and volunteer work or hobbies should be considered.

11. Are teenagers less vulnerable to workplace chemical exposures because they are young and healthy? When we were young, we worked without all these protections.

Risks of exposures can be small or life-threatening, depending on the chemical. Teenagers and children are just as vulnerable to enclosed space exposures as older workers. Theoretically, if a chemical becomes less toxic when broken down by the body, and teenagers break down chemicals better or faster than adults, then its effects could be less toxic for a young worker. If the chemical after it is broken down is poisonous, however, teenagers could be at increased risk. Because one is unlikely to know in advance which situation is the case for any given chemical, testing the situation may involve risking illness or death. Thus, protection from exposure is always the best approach.

12. Are teenagers more vulnerable than adults to toxins in the work environment because their systems (especially immune systems) are not yet fully developed?

Adolescents may be more vulnerable in some respects but not because of their immune systems. The immune system is essentially fully developed by adolescence, so it is not likely to be more vulnerable.

If we know, however, that an exposure is hazardous for adults, we should assume that it is likely to be at least as hazardous for adolescents and protect them from that exposure. Exposure to potentially cancer-causing substances and to substances that may produce birth defects may create increased risk for adolescents because they have more future years. There may be higher risks of early life exposure to substances (especially those that cause cancer) associated with diseases that occur only after a long time has passed. If a substance accumulates in the body over time and the effects are related to how much a person is exposed to, teen workers may be at risk because their exposure started earlier in life. It is possible that exposure to a cancer-causing chemical during the rapid growth period of adolescence may increase cancer risk. Given that adolescence is a time of changes to the endocrine system, there may be increased vulnerability to chemicals (including certain pesticides) that can disrupt the endocrine system. Because adolescents are of childbearing age, immediate and longer-term reproductive effects of chemicals are potentially of concern.

13. Is it safe for a teenager who is still growing to do manual labor with heavy equipment?

Current knowledge about occupational back injury and about overuse injuries among young gymnasts and baseball players suggests that periods of rapid growth may put an individual at increased risk of severe and chronic injuries to the bones and soft tissues, especially if there are too many repetitions of a movement. This has implications for farmwork, cashier work, and any work with repetitive motion.

Chapter 11

Navigating Your Child's Health Care

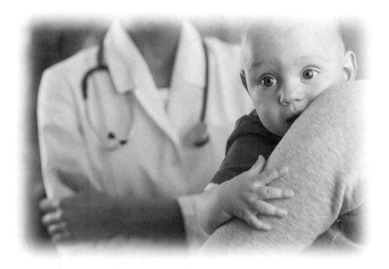

Blood and Other Testing for Environmental Toxicants

1. **Cadmium was measured in my child's blood, and the result was higher than normal. I am told that cadmium is a cancer-causing chemical. Does this mean my child will get cancer?**

   Many chemicals have been classified as carcinogens (meaning that they cause cancer) according to studies of animals that were given high doses of the chemical, often over long periods, or workers who were exposed to large amounts of the chemical, usually over many years. The likelihood of developing cancer is affected by a person's genetics, life habits (including smoking), diet, and environmental exposures. Healthy eating that includes foods high in levels of vitamins, antioxidants, and fiber, along with avoiding chemicals that cause cancer, helps reduce the likelihood of cancer.

   To prevent a child's exposure to cadmium, stop smoking and eliminate smoke exposure in your home and car. Cigarette smoke is a well-known source of cadmium because tobacco plants take up cadmium found in the soil. A child also may be exposed to cadmium after swallowing cadmium-containing jewelry or biting, sucking, or mouthing such jewelry.

2. **The laboratory staff reported my son's blood level of mercury as being above the reference range. What does this mean?**

   The laboratory reference range is usually the range of values that were measured by that laboratory in either 95% or 97.5% of patient samples. If the child's blood level is lower than the 95th percentile for mercury, the interpretation is that the child's exposure is similar to the general population exposure. A mercury result higher than the 95th percentile means that only 5% of the general population has higher values and greater exposure to mercury. If your son's mercury level is high, consider whether he ate mercury-contaminated fish within 2 to 3 days before the blood was drawn; this could be the reason for his high mercury levels.

3. **Should my child's blood be tested for perfluoroalkylated and polyfluoroalkylated substances (PFAS)?**

Although a number of perfluoroalkylated and poly-fluoroalkylated substances (PFAS) can be measured in serum, the testing requires specialized laboratory staff and complex technology that are not available in clinical laboratories. Because the results do not guide medical therapy or predict future health effects, serum PFAS measurements are not generally available outside of research studies. In communities in which contaminated drinking water was discovered, serum PFAS measurements were part of the public health response determining the extent of exposure. However, routine measurements of serum PFAS are not recommended because few laboratories measure PFAS, the tests are costly and unlikely to be covered by insurance, and the results do not provide information that can help a doctor treat your child. If you are concerned, contact your pediatrician with any questions you might have.

4. I paid a lot of money to have blood tests done on my child to identify the presence of harmful chemicals. The results showed that my child has harmful chemicals in his body and I want them removed. How do I get these harmful chemicals out of his body?

Unless your pediatrician or other health care professional ordered the test and was involved in the decision-making process, these tests may have been unnecessary. Your pediatrician may not be able to interpret or make recommendations based on these results for several reasons. Many of these tests are not performed in certified laboratories and reference (normal) ranges are not available; therefore, the results are not interpretable. In addition, finding a chemical in the body does not mean that the chemical causes a health problem.

Many of the chemicals may already have been deactivated (metabolized) and eliminated from the body. Some chemicals are very slowly eliminated from the body. Identifying and eliminating sources of the child's exposure to hazardous chemicals is the best course of action.

Many therapies promoted to speed elimination of chemicals from the body are unproven or even dangerous. Consult with your pediatrician to determine if your child has any health problems that may be related to the chemicals identified by laboratory testing. If such metals as lead, mercury, and cadmium were among the measurements, chelation therapy to remove any of these substances is not recommended and may be harmful. Chelation therapy is a method used to bond chemicals and remove them from the blood. The only US Food and Drug

Administration–approved indication for oral chelation therapy is for blood lead levels greater than 45 micrograms per deciliter. Other uses of chelation are unproven, experimental, and potentially hazardous.

5. I have heard that laboratories can measure many harmful chemicals in my child's blood. Can my child's pediatrician order these tests?

It is not a good idea to test for chemicals because not enough studies have been conducted to understand what the results mean. Very few chemicals can be measured and interpreted accurately. Your pediatrician will use scientifically proven practices when ordering, interpreting, and making recommendations based on laboratory tests to assess for exposures. Otherwise, interpretation of the results is usually not possible because information on reference (normal) values and levels that may be linked to harmful effects is not available. In addition, the presence of a chemical in the body does not mean that the chemical causes a health problem.

6. What is the blood lead reference value?

The reference value is used to identify children with elevated blood lead levels—that is, the top 2.5% of blood lead levels. The reference value is based on the 97.5th percentile of blood lead levels in American children aged 1 to 5 years, measured as part of a large national survey of Americans. The current reference value, 5 micrograms per deciliter (mcg/dL) of blood, comes from blood lead levels measured from 2007 through 2010. The reference value can be recalculated every 4 years as new blood lead data become available. Children with elevated blood lead levels should be monitored but do not need chelation therapy unless the blood lead level is higher than

45 mcg/dL. The most important step is to find out where the lead is coming from by looking for lead paint hazards in housing and removing your child from the hazard. It is also important to give your child healthy foods to reduce lead absorption.

7. Can toxic chemicals or metals be reliably measured by taking a sample of hair?

Hair samples have been used to measure environmental chemicals and metals, but the results cannot distinguish metals in the hair from those deposited from external contaminants. Hair mercury has been measured in research studies, using strict rules that guide the collection of samples. Typical medical laboratories do not have standard processes for collecting and preparing hair specimens and analyzing them. The wide range of hair treatments, shampoos, and conditioners that are used by Americans may contain metals or chemicals that leave deposits on the hair or may remove chemicals or metals from the hair. Thus, hair measurement is not a reliable indicator of what is inside a person's body. In addition, the results cannot be compared to conventional results, such as blood or urine concentrations. Your pediatrician may not be able to interpret the results or make recommendations because the results may not be reliable. In addition, no evidence shows that testing of hair for environmental chemicals or metals helps to diagnose or treat autism spectrum disorder (for short, ASD).

8. What can I do or give my daughter to help get rid of the perfluoroalkylated and polyfluoroalkylated substances (PFAS) in her body?

In the body, perfluorooctane sulfonate (for short, PFOS), perfluorooctanoic acid (for short, PFOA), and perfluorohexane sulfonate (for short, PFHxS)

are mostly bound to albumin and other serum proteins, but some of the chemicals may be stored in the
liver and possibly other organs. These chemicals are
not broken down by the body, and they are gotten
rid of in the urine very slowly. There is no known
medication or process to speed the body's natural
mechanism for getting rid of perfluoroalkylated and
polyfluoroalkylated substances (PFAS) in urine or to
remove them from the blood.

Dental Issues

9. **I am debating getting dental sealants for my
   twins, but I am concerned that sealants contain
   bisphenol A (BPA). I read about concerns that
   BPA may have effects on the endocrine system.
   Are dental sealants safe?**

   Dental sealants play an important role in preventing tooth decay and cavities and, for this reason,
   are routinely recommended. Talk with your dentist.
   Techniques, such as using a pumice stone to wipe
   off the uncured layer of sealant after applying it, along
   with having children rinse with water and then spit,
   have been found to reduce bisphenol A (BPA) exposure during the application process. Bisphenol A–free
   sealants also are available.

10. **Should my child have nonmercury fillings? Or,
    should mercury fillings be replaced?**

    Mercury fillings (amalgams) are a durable material
    for filling cavities. There is no scientific evidence that
    this commonly used dental material causes harm to a
    child, although a small amount of mercury exposure
    may occur from the presence of dental fillings. It is
    not necessary to replace fillings just because of the

mercury content; furthermore, the removal process may weaken the tooth.

X-rays

11. How many X-ray exams are safe for my child?

Your child's pediatrician will take into account the benefit of X-ray examinations (exams) and the risk in diagnosing and monitoring your child's health condition. In most situations, the benefit of X-ray exams is more worthwhile than the very small risk. Because the radiation doses from certain diagnostic procedures—for example, computed tomography (CT) scans—are high, pediatricians often prefer to order radiologic exams (such as ultrasound or magnetic resonance imaging) that do not emit ionizing radiation, if the exam is appropriate for your child's situation. Your pediatrician will order radiologic exams emitting ionizing radiation only when necessary and will check to ensure that CT scan operators use settings appropriate for children.

12. Will X-ray exams of my child affect future grandchildren?

It is highly unlikely that an individual's X-ray examinations (exams) would affect future children or grandchildren.

Specific Health Conditions

Asthma

13. Why is asthma on the increase?

Scientists and public health officials are concerned by the apparent increase in the number of people who have asthma. The explanation for the increase has not been found but seems most likely to be related to a complex combination of factors, including increased exposure to environmental allergens and irritants indoors; increased exposure to complex environmental pollutants, such as secondhand tobacco smoke, diesel exhaust, and irritant gases during infancy; genetic susceptibility; delayed maturation of immune responses because of changes in exposure to infection and infectious products; dietary factors; and stress and poverty. Emerging evidence from scientific studies suggests that being exposed to air pollution in the long term and living close to high traffic areas may cause some cases of asthma, especially in those people who are genetically prone to developing asthma.

14. Is there good scientific evidence that exposure to secondhand smoke is linked to asthma in young children?

Yes. There is enough evidence showing a strong association between exposure to secondhand smoke and the development of asthma or wheezing in young children.

15. My child recently was diagnosed with asthma. Should I get an air filtration system for his room or the whole house?

Avoid room humidifiers and keep central furnace system humidification below 50% during winter months. Filters on central forced-air systems and furnaces should be changed regularly, according to manufacturers' recommendations. The Minimum Efficiency Reporting Value (MERV) rating is the standard method for comparing the efficiency of air filters. The higher the MERV rating, the better the filter is at removing particles from the air. Upgrading to a medium-efficiency filter (rated at 20%–50% efficiency at removing particles between 0.3 and 10 micrometers [MERV 8–12]) will improve air quality and is economical. Electrostatic filters/precipitators in central furnace and air-conditioning systems may be beneficial for airborne particles (such as cat allergens). Avoid the use of air cleaners (usually labeled as electrostatic) that generate ozone.

Room high-efficiency particulate air (for short, HEPA) filters also may be beneficial. However, they only work in a single room, and the noise generated may not be acceptable. Preferably, they should be used in the child's bedroom.

16. Should I get a special vacuum cleaner to avoid triggering an asthma attack in my child when I clean the house?

Other methods to reduce allergen exposure are more beneficial. However, an efficient vacuum cleaner that avoids driving allergens back into the air may be useful for removing allergens, especially from hard surfaces. Leakage of allergen is minimized in vacuum cleaners that incorporate a double-thickness bag and have tight-fitting junctions within the cleaner; a high-efficiency particulate air (for short, HEPA) filter is not always necessary, depending on vacuum design. Unfortunately, there is no certification process to guide consumers.

17. What can I do in my house to prevent asthma attacks from occurring?

Quit smoking if you smoke, and eliminate exposures to secondhand smoke by making sure your home and car are kept smoke-free. Reduce dust mites, cockroaches, and home dampness or molds. Consider removing carpeting. Remove pets to which the child demonstrates specific allergy. If removing the pet is not possible, keep pets out of the bedroom and routinely perform allergen reduction measures (vacuuming and minimizing reservoirs of dander, such as pillows). If the pet is not removed, it will be nearly impossible to avoid exposure. Consider using a vacuum cleaner that is efficient at cleaning and avoids driving allergens back into the air, such as one equipped with a high-efficiency particulate air (for short, HEPA) filter.

18. I have heard that antioxidants can prevent asthma in my child. Should I give her a supplement?

Studies of vitamins and antioxidants have not shown consistent results regarding preventing the development of asthma or improving asthma control.

19. My child has asthma, but I don't have any mold, animals, or insects in my home that I can see. Could she have an allergy to dust mites?

If your child has asthma and allergy symptoms, allergy testing will typically be done. Dust mites are common indoor allergens and will be part of the allergy test panel. They are a known trigger of asthma and there is evidence that avoiding dust mites improves asthma outcomes. Allergy shots may help patients with asthma who are sensitized to dust mites. Allergy testing may include a skin test or a blood test.

Cancer

20. Are rates of childhood cancer increasing?

Yes. Rates of childhood cancer (in children and adolescents younger than 15 years) increased 38% from 1975 to 2014 in the United States. For leukemia, the most common childhood cancer, there was a 42% increase in incidence rates; increases were greatest for Hispanic children. For brain cancer and other nervous system cancers, incidence increased in the 1980s because of improvements in diagnostic procedures and changes in classification. Rates were stable from 1987 to 2014. Among children, adolescents, and young adults (younger than 20), non-Hodgkin lymphoma rates increased, whereas Hodgkin lymphoma rates decreased over the same period.

21. What steps can I take to prevent cancer in my child?

Although the causes of many childhood cancers are unknown, there is consistent evidence that the chance of getting childhood leukemia increases with exposures to pesticides, solvents, traffic-related air pollution, and smoking by a child's father. Therefore, it is a good idea to limit these exposures during pregnancy and throughout the child's life.

Breastfeeding; folic acid supplementation during pregnancy; and a healthy diet, which includes limited or no consumption of cured/smoked meats and cured/smoked fish; and frequent intake of fruits and vegetables have been shown to reduce the chances of getting childhood leukemia. Children and teenagers should be encouraged not to smoke, use electronic cigarettes or similar devices, or use smokeless tobacco products. You should quit smoking; if you keep smoking, you should never smoke indoors or in the car to prevent others from being exposed to secondhand smoke.

Too much exposure to ultraviolet (for short, UV) radiation from the sun or from tanning beds can cause skin cancer later in life. Children should be encouraged to wear clothing and hats and to use sunscreen when outdoors so that they do not become sunburned. Teenagers should not be allowed to tan in tanning salons or other venues, such as health clubs, that may have tanning beds. Other important measures to prevent cancer include testing your home for radon and making sure no asbestos in the home is crumbling.

22. Our child has leukemia and was exposed to power lines. Could this have caused the leukemia?

Pinpointing the cause of your child's leukemia is currently beyond the ability of science. Even when scientists are convinced that a factor, such as ionizing radiation, can cause childhood leukemia, it is impossible to be certain whether a particular case of leukemia was caused by radiation. It is even more problematic to determine how much the electric and magnetic fields from power lines contribute to any illness. This is because there is only weak scientific evidence showing that these fields may cause harm to humans.

23. Is my child's leukemia attributable to past radiation exposures?

There is no way to determine this for an individual child. Illnesses induced by radiation cannot be distinguished from illnesses in the general population. The relationship can only be established by large studies of the population that show a higher incidence among a group of people who got high doses of radiation (such as atomic bomb survivors).

24. My sister has thyroid cancer and receives radioiodine as treatment. Is it safe for my kids to be around her right now?

The American Thyroid Association Taskforce on Radioiodine Safety has developed recommendations that comply with Nuclear Regulatory Commission regulations and guidelines put forth by the National Council on Radiation Protection and Measurements. The recommendations depend on the dose of radioiodine that a patient receives. During the day, your sister should stay at least 6 feet (2 meters) apart from children and women for 1 day, regardless of how much radioiodine she received.

Any patient receiving radioiodine should sleep in a separate bed from pregnant partners, children, or infants for 6 to 21 days following treatment of thyroid cancer and 15 to 23 days following treatment of an overactive thyroid gland (hyperthyroidism).

25. If my husband receives myocardial perfusion testing with thallium, does he need to stay away from our children?

Myocardial perfusion testing is done to determine if parts of the heart muscle are not receiving enough blood. During the testing, a liquid with a small amount of thallium is injected into a vein. The thallium contains a small amount of radioactivity. There are not many studies on the effect of the dose of thallium and contact with others. However, one study showed that at a distance of 3 feet (1 meter), there is no exposure above background levels of radiation.

26. Why did neuroblastoma develop in my 3-month-old child?

We do not know why. We do know that damage (an alteration) to DNA occurs at a specific location in one chromosome in children with neuroblastoma, but we do not know what causes the mutation. Mutations may occur during normal reshuffling of genetic material. Usually, the damage is repaired and cancer does not develop, but unfortunately, this defense is sometimes not enough.

27. Our cat has been sick. Could the cat have caused my child's leukemia?

There is no evidence that pets transmit cancer to humans. Cats develop a similar disease caused by a virus, which they can transmit to other cats but not to humans. The same is true of chickens and cattle, in which a leukemia-like disease is caused by a virus.

28. Several children in our neighborhood have cancer. Could it be caused by the same thing?

Although most environmental causes of cancer in humans have been first recognized by the occurrence of a cluster of cases, such discoveries are infrequent and generally involve rare cancers attributable to heavy exposures to a cancer-causing substance. The many types of cancer (more than 80) give rise to thousands of random clusters each year in the United States in neighborhoods, schools, social clubs, sports teams, and other groups of people. By focusing on the location of cases, an otherwise random clustering of cases may seem to be unusual. To establish a cause, however, more evidence than a neighborhood cluster is needed, including a "dose-response effect" (the bigger the dose, the more frequent the effect) and determining whether scientific information about this cancer cluster fits with other knowledge about the cancer. In most neighborhood clusters, there are many different types of cancers and many different causes, rather than a single cause.

29. Can my child with cancer give my other children cancer?

Cancer is not transmitted from one child to another. Occasionally, a genetic tendency to specific cancers is transmitted from parents to children, which may have implications for other children in the family.

For example, retinoblastoma (a rare cancer of the eye) runs in families. Usually, signs of a tendency to inherited cancers can be detected in your family history. For children at risk, early detection and treatment can improve survival and well-being. Thus, few children die of retinoblastoma today.

30. A member of our household smokes. Could that be the cause of my child's cancer?

There is increasing evidence that a father's smoking (but not a mother's smoking) before and during the pregnancy increases the risk of childhood leukemia in offspring. Cancers in children and adolescents younger than 15 years generally are of a different microscopic category from adult cigarette-induced cancers, and no evidence currently exists that the childhood cancers can start by being exposed to secondhand smoke. On the other hand, adult cancers, such as lung cancer, leukemia, and lymphoma, have been associated with exposure to maternal smoking that occurs before the child reaches age 10 years.

31. Is it possible that the medicine I took during pregnancy started my child's cancer?

Diethylstilbestrol (DES) is the only known medication given to pregnant mothers that is associated with increased cancer risk among their children. It has not been used since the 1970s and was associated primarily with cancer of the vagina in young women whose mothers took DES during pregnancy. Other drugs commonly used during pregnancy have not been shown to cause cancer in the offspring. Drugs shown to present a risk of either birth defects or a possible risk of cancer are generally avoided during pregnancy.

32. I have heard that peanut butter may cause cancer. Is this true?

Peanuts can be contaminated with molds that produce aflatoxins, which are toxic chemicals that cause cancer. The US Food and Drug Administration allows aflatoxins at low levels in nuts, seeds, and legumes because aflatoxins are considered "unavoidable contaminants." If a particular batch of peanut butter is tested and the concentration of aflatoxin is over the action level, it will be subject to a recall. Aflatoxins have been shown to increase the risk of liver cancer in adults; however, there is no evidence of a link with childhood cancers.

33. Does living near a nuclear power plant increase my child's risk of cancer?

One study in Germany showed that children younger than 5 with leukemia were more than twice as likely as a comparison group of children to live within 3.1 miles (5 kilometers) of a nuclear power plant. It is not clear whether this association means that living nearer to a nuclear power plant causes leukemia.

Additional studies are needed to clarify the risk of living near a nuclear power plant.

Developmental Disabilities

34. My 3-year-old son was recently diagnosed with autism spectrum disorder (ASD). I wonder if chelation for metal poisoning might help him. I met some other parents who say that they felt it helped their children. Should I consider this? What are the risks?

Medicine does not yet offer curative treatments for autism. Research shows no association between exposure to metals and autism. Chelation (a method that bonds chemicals and removes them from blood) is risky and not recommended.

Children, including children with autism spectrum disorder (ASD), continue to develop, and it is possible that improvements in behaviors may seem as if they follow a specific treatment such as chelation, when the improvements may actually be due to development. Scientifically established behavioral therapies have been associated with improved outcomes for young children with ASD.

35. I've heard that vaccines cause autism.

In the past, some people were concerned about whether mercury found in some vaccines caused any health effects. Some influenza vaccines contain small amounts of thimerosal (a substance that contains ethyl mercury) as a preservative to prevent bacterial overgrowth. Thimerosal does not stay in the body a long time, so it does not build up and reach harmful levels. When thimerosal enters the body, it breaks down to ethyl mercury and thiosalicylate, which are readily eliminated. Measles, mumps, and rubella (for short, MMR) vaccines do not and never did contain thimerosal. Varicella (chickenpox), inactivated polio-virus (for short, IPV), and pneumococcal conjugate vaccines also have never contained thimerosal. Influenza (flu) vaccines are currently available in both thimerosal-containing (for multidose vaccine vials) and thimerosal-free versions. If you are concerned, ask your doctor for the thimerosal-free version.

Vaccines are among the safest medical products in use. All children should be vaccinated on time so they are protected from vaccine-preventable diseases. Children are harmed from these illnesses and doctors are trying to prevent these diseases. Results from many research studies show no connection between vaccines and autism. Review the Vaccine Information Statements from the Centers for Disease Control and Prevention (www.cdc.gov/vaccines/hcp/vis/index. html) so you can learn more about the vaccines.

36. I have been told that my child has a short attention span and that he frequently is inattentive in class. The teacher has suggested psychological testing. My child is fine at home. Could these problems be related to chemical exposure at school?

A thorough evaluation of your child's difficulty and appropriate testing are initial steps in dealing with this problem. Sources of potential environmental contam-ination cited in schools include cleaning agents, art supplies (such as glues, markers, or aerosol sprays), pesticides, and diesel exhaust fumes from school buses. Dust and molds also are sources of indoor air pollution. Symptoms in one setting only (the school) may suggest that something in the school environment may be the problem. Often, when asked, other students and teachers in a school with poor indoor air quality or other environmental hazards will report similar health concerns.

Obesity

37. My child is overweight and has acanthosis nigricans (a darkening of certain parts of skin) with a high serum insulin level. Do you think she is deficient in chromium? Should her level be measured?

There is no known correlation between chromium deficiency and insulin resistance; therefore, obtaining a chromium level in blood or urine would not be helpful. In addition, it is difficult to collect a blood specimen without some chromium contamination from the stainless-steel needle used to obtain the blood specimen.

38. I am concerned about my son's weight. He continues to gain weight despite my efforts to help him eat healthier. I have heard news stories about chemicals in the food supply (such as bisphenol A [for short, BPA] lining cans or phthalates in food packaging) and wonder if there is more I can do to make healthy food choices. Is there?

The best way is to eliminate sugar-sweetened beverages and increase the servings of fruits and vegetables he eats every day. You should also reduce high-calorie/high-fat foods, decrease the number of times you eat food outside the home, encourage small portions, ensure that he eats breakfast every day, encourage family meals and healthy snacks, and provide lots of whole grains, lean proteins, and water.

To reduce your son's exposure to chemicals in foods, choose fresh foods over processed foods. Consider choosing organic foods when possible, especially for foods that a child eats often that may be high in levels of pesticides. Readily available guides can help you identify conventional (nonorganic) foods that are low in levels of pesticides. One such resource is the Environmental Working Group's annual listing of the Clean Fifteen and Dirty Dozen (conventional fruits and vegetables either lowest or highest in levels of pesticides). Children should eat a variety of foods, especially fruits and vegetables (organic or nonorganic—see www.choosemyplate.gov/resources/myplate-10-tips), and drink mostly water instead of sugary drinks.

Resources include

- Environmental Working Group's 2020 Shopper's Guide to Pesticides in Produce (www.ewg.org/foodnews/dirty_dozen_list.php#.WmY2SrynGUk)

- Pediatric Environmental Health Specialty Units *Consumer Guide: Phthalates and Bisphenol* (www.pehsu.net/_Library/facts/bpapatients_factsheet03-2014.pdf)

- US Department of Agriculture "MyPlate Tip Sheets" (www.choosemyplate.gov/resources/myplate-10-tips)

39. I have been told my child is obese. I am worried about the lack of fresh, affordable fruits and vegetables in my neighborhood and also worry about my child's safety while playing in local parks. What can I do?

Children should receive their fruits and vegetables in any form that is available. Frozen and canned (without endocrine-disrupting chemical [for short, EDC] liners) can be good alternatives when fresh produce is not available. Some families who qualify might benefit from their local Special Supplemental Nutrition Program for Women, Infants, and Children (WIC) and local food bank. Other local resources may be available. Free or low-cost physical activity resources, such as after-school programs and summer camps, may be available and can significantly increase the amount of time your child spends outdoors and in active play. Local public health agencies and community-based organizations often have information on additional resources for children. You may want to voice your concerns at local community board meetings or Parent-Teacher Association meetings or by calling or writing to your local government representatives. The American Academy of Pediatrics has information for parents and other caregivers; for more information, please visit www.healthychildren.org and search for "healthy lifestyle."

Resources include

- Special Supplemental Nutrition Program for WIC (www.fns.usda.gov/wic/women-infants-and-children-wic)

- Supplemental Nutrition Assistance Program (for short, SNAP) (www.fns.usda.gov/snap/supplemental nutrition-assistance-program-snap)

- *Children & Nature* infographic (www.neefusa.org/resource/children-and-nature-infographic)

- *Children's Health & Urban Parks* infographic (http://envhealthcenters.usc.edu/infographics/infographic-childrens-health-urban-parks)

- National Farmers Market Directory (www.ams.usda.gov/local-food-directories/farmersmarkets)

Chapter 12

The Big Green Picture

Saving People and the Planet

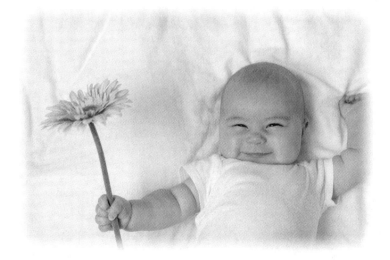

1. **I am concerned about the environment and have read that some sunscreen ingredients are washed off from the skin into ocean water and may contribute to bleaching of coral reefs. Is this true?**

   Certain sunscreen ingredients, such as oxybenzone, may contribute significantly to coral reef bleaching and therefore may be hazardous to coral reefs. Other reports suggest that climate change is the main hazard to coral reefs. More research is needed in this area. You should take steps needed to prevent sunburning and other overexposure to the sun to lessen your chance of developing skin cancer.

2. **Is it OK to flush unused prescription drugs down the toilet?**

   Residues of birth control pills, antidepressants, painkillers, shampoos, and many other drugs and personal care products have been found in water, in trace amounts. These chemicals are flushed into rivers from sewage treatment plants or leach into groundwater from septic systems. The discovery of these substances in water probably reflects better sensing technology. The health effects, if any, from exposure to these substances in water are not yet known.

   In many cases, these chemicals enter water when people excrete them or wash them away in the shower. Some chemicals, however, are flushed or washed down the drain when people discard outdated or unused drugs.

   Prescription or over-the-counter medications should not be flushed down the toilet or poured down a sink unless patient information material specifically states that it is safe to do so.

(See www.fda.gov/drugs/resourcesforyou/consumers/
buyingusingmedicinesafely/ensuringsafeuseofmedicine/
safedisposalofmedicines/ucm186187.htm.)

If no disposal instructions are given on the prescription drug labeling, then use the following US Food and Drug Administration guidelines to dispose of these products properly and to prevent harm from unintentional exposure or intentional misuse after they are no longer needed:

- Follow any specific disposal instructions on the prescription drug labeling or patient information that accompanies the medicine. Do not flush medicines down the sink or toilet unless this information specifically instructs you to do so.

- Take advantage of programs that allow the public to take unused drugs to a central location for proper disposal. Call your local law enforcement agencies to see if they sponsor medicine take-back programs in your community. Contact your city's or county government's household trash and recycling service to learn about medication disposal options and guidelines for your area.

- Transfer unused medicines to collectors registered with the Drug Enforcement Administration (DEA). Authorized sites may be retail, hospital or clinic pharmacies, and law enforcement locations. Some offer mail-back programs or collection receptacles ("drop-boxes"). Visit the DEA's Web site (www.deadiversion.usdoj.gov/drug_disposal/index.html) or call 1-800-882-9539 for more information and to find an authorized collector (www.deadiversion.usdoj.gov/pubdispsearch/spring/main?execution=e1s1) in your community.

If no disposal instructions are given on the prescription drug labeling and no take-back program is available in your area, throw the drugs in the household trash following these steps:

1. Remove them from their original containers and mix them with an undesirable substance, such as used coffee grounds, dirt or kitty litter (this makes the drug less appealing to children and pets, and unrecognizable to people who may intentionally go through the trash seeking drugs).

2. Place the mixture in a sealable bag, empty can, or other container to prevent the drug from leaking or breaking out of a garbage bag.

3. Have any states or countries set standards for electric and magnetic fields?

Lack of knowledge has prevented scientists from strongly recommending any health-based regulations regarding electric fields and magnetic fields. The International Agency for Research on Cancer recommends that policy makers establish guidelines for electric and magnetic field exposures for both the general public and workers and that low-cost measures of reducing exposure be considered.

Several states have adopted regulations governing transmission line-generated 60-Hertz fields. The initial concern was the risk of electric shock from strong electric fields (measured in kilovolts [kV] per meter). Some states, such as Florida and New York, have adopted regulations that prevent new lines from exceeding the fields at the edge of the current right-of-way. The California Department of Education requires that new schools be built at certain distances from transmission lines. These distances, 100 feet (ft)

(30 meters [m]) for 100-kV power lines and 250 ft (76 m) for 345-kV power lines, were chosen on the basis of the estimate that electric fields would have reached the background level at these distances.

All of the current regulations relate to transmission lines, and no state has adopted regulations that govern distribution lines, substations, appliances, or other sources of electric and magnetic fields.

4. **Should I be concerned about proposals to add methylcyclopentadienyl manganese tricarbonyl (MMT) to gasoline as an antiknock agent?**

Yes. Manganese is toxic to the nervous system. This manganese additive is not used currently in US gasoline. It was used in Canada to improve octane rating and as an antiknock agent but has since been phased out. A few other countries, such as Australia and South Africa, permit the use of methylcyclopentadienyl manganese tricarbonyl (MMT). Toxic effects on the nervous system have been seen at high- and low-dose exposures and span the range from tremors and other problems associated with Parkinson disease at high exposures to subtle behavior problems. Permitting the addition of MMT to the US gasoline supply would not be prudent. This could increase the risk of widespread mild nervous system problems.

5. **How can national governments reduce population exposure to persistent organic pollutants (POPs)?**

National governments can reduce exposures to persistent organic pollutants (POPs) by curtailing and banning their manufacture and use by joining the Stockholm Convention on Persistent Organic Pollutants, an international treaty signed in 2001 that aims to eliminate or restrict production and use of POPs. Other steps include controlling industrial sources of environmental release of POPs, controlling their release from municipal landfills and hazardous waste sites, requiring incineration of polychlorinated biphenyl (for short, PCB)–contaminated waste materials at temperatures over 1,562 degrees Fahrenheit (850 degrees Celsius) in specially constructed incinerators in order to prevent formation of dioxins, and establishing and enforcing strict programs for monitoring of these chemicals in the food supply.

6. How can state and local governments reduce population exposure to persistent organic pollutants (POPs)?

Persistent organic pollutants (POPs) are a large group of different chemicals that stay in the body and environment for long periods of time. State and local governments can reduce exposures by controlling commercial sources of release and securing landfills. Local governments can control the spread of polychlorinated biphenyls (PCBs) (a POP commonly used in the past) in school environments by requiring timely removal of all PCB-containing fluorescent light ballasts. Parents can accelerate this process through citizen action.

7. Will the US Environmental Protection Agency (EPA) ban the use of chlorpyrifos, an organophosphate pesticide?

The US EPA banned chlorpyrifos use in homes in 2000 except in select cases, including when chlorpyrifos is contained in ant and roach bait products. The US EPA also banned its use on some crops, such as tomatoes, and limited its use on other crops, including apples, grapes, and citrus fruits. A total ban has not yet happened. The US EPA extended the timeline for its review of a total ban until 2022.

8. **Why is there controversy over bisphenol A (BPA) (a chemical that makes plastics rigid)?**

Bisphenol A (BPA) affects endocrine functions in animals. The controversy arises because there are few studies showing harmful effects in infants or children. There is concern, however, that children are rapidly growing and developing and may, therefore, be especially susceptible to chemicals such as BPA. Additional research studies and reviews by the US Food and Drug Administration may determine what level of exposure to BPA might cause similar effects in humans.

9. **Is anything being done to advocate for safety testing of chemicals before they are put on the market? It appears that we are always finding possible and actual hazards of new chemicals but not until after they have been released into the environment.**

The American Academy of Pediatrics and other organizations strongly advocate for protecting children, pregnant women, and the general population from the hazards of chemicals before the chemicals are marketed.

The Precautionary Principle states that those who wish to implement or sell a product, including chemicals and products containing chemicals, should have to prove that it is safe rather than wait for scientific proof that it causes harm.

Many precautionary tools are available, including bans and restricted use, substitution, redesign, and improved materials management. Some bans, such as banning lead from gasoline, paint, and children's toys and jewelry, are appropriate. In other situations, restrictions or substitutions may be enough.

10. Doesn't the Precautionary Principle stifle innovation?

Because the Precautionary Principle explicitly requires exploring alternative technologies and solutions by experts and the public, it can enhance innovation. For example, developing renewable, clean energy to satisfy increased energy demands would be preferred over creating more coal-fired power plants. Using pigments that are biodegradable, are nontoxic, and do not contain metals would be preferred over older pigments containing known cancer-causing chemicals and heavy metals.

Appendix

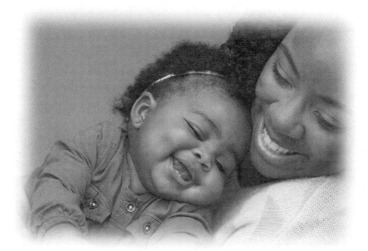

Resources

The American Academy of Pediatrics has not reviewed the material on these websites. Inclusion in this list does not imply endorsement.

The material in this appendix is organized as follows:

- US federal and state governments
- Non-US governments including the World Health Organization (WHO)
- Nongovernmental organizations including
  - Children's Environmental Health and Disease Prevention Research Centers
  - Pediatric Environmental Health Specialty Units (PEHSUs)

Organization	Contact Information
US Federal and State Governments	
FEDERAL AGENCIES	
Agency for Toxic Substances and Disease Registry (ATSDR) 1600 Clifton Rd NE Stop E-28 Atlanta, GA 30333	www.atsdr.cdc.gov
– ATSDR Toxicological Profiles	www.atsdr.cdc.gov/toxprofiles/index.asp
– ATSDR Regional Offices	www.atsdr.cdc.gov/dro
National Cancer Institute	www.cancer.gov 1-800-4-CANCER (1-800-422-6237) Surveillance, Epidemiology, and End Results (SEER) Program: www.seer.cancer.gov
National Center for Environmental Health (NCEH) Centers for Disease Control and Prevention (CDC) 4770 Buford Hwy NE Atlanta, GA 30341-3717	www.cdc.gov/nceh

– NCEH National Asthma Control Program	www.cdc.gov/nceh/information/asthma.htm
– NCEH Childhood Lead Poisoning Prevention Program	www.cdc.gov/nceh/lead
– *National Report on Human Exposure to Environmental Chemicals*	www.cdc.gov/exposurereport
National Institute for Occupational Safety and Health (NIOSH)	www.cdc.gov/niosh/homepage.html
– NIOSH "Young Worker Safety and Health"	www.cdc.gov/niosh/topics/youth
National Institute of Environmental Health Sciences (NIEHS) PO Box 12233 Research Triangle Park, NC 27709	www.niehs.nih.gov
– National Toxicology Program (NTP)	www.ntp.niehs.nih.gov
– *Environmental Health Perspectives*	ehp.niehs.nih.gov
– "Children's Environmental Health"	www.niehs.nih.gov/health/topics/population/children/index.cfm
– NIEHS Superfund Research Program	www.niehs.nih.gov/research/supported/centers/srp/index.cfm

Organization	Contact Information
National Institutes of Health (NIH) 9000 Rockville Pike Bethesda, MD 20892	nih.gov
– Drugs and Lactation Database (LactMed)	www.ncbi.nlm.nih.gov/books/NBK501922
– Tox Town	toxtown.nlm.nih.gov
Office of Lead Hazard Control and Healthy Homes US Department of Housing and Urban Development 451 7th St SW Washington, DC 20410	www.hud.gov/program_offices/healthy_homes
Smokefree.gov	Smokefree.gov 1-800-QUIT-NOW (1-800-784-8669)
US Consumer Product Safety Commission (CPSC) 4330 East West Hwy Bethesda, MD 20814	www.cpsc.gov

US Department of Agriculture	www.usda.gov
– Food Safety and Inspection Service 1400 Independence Ave SW Washington, DC 20250	"Food Safety Education": www.fsis.usda.gov/wps/portal/fsis/topics/food-safety-education
US Environmental Protection Agency (EPA) 1200 Pennsylvania Ave NW Washington, DC 20460	www.epa.gov
– US EPA Office of Children's Health Protection Protecting Children's Environmental Health	www.epa.gov/children
– US EPA Office of Pesticide Programs	Pesticides: www.epa.gov/pesticides Poison Control Center: 1-800-222-1222
– US EPA Office of Air and Radiation	"About the Office of Air and Radiation (OAR)": www.epa.gov/oar Indoor air: www.epa.gov/indoor-air-quality-iaq Creating Healthy Indoor Air Quality in Schools: www.epa.gov/iaq-schools AirNow—ground-level ozone: www.airnow.gov Healthy School Environments: www.epa.gov/schools/healthyseat/index.html

Organization	Contact Information
US Environmental Protection Agency (EPA) *(continued)*	
– US EPA Endocrine Disruption	www.epa.gov/endocrine-disruption
– US EPA Office of Emergency Management	www.epa.gov/emergency-response/national-response-center 1-800-424-8802
– US EPA Office of Ground Water and Drinking Water	www.epa.gov/aboutepa/about-office-water#ground
– US EPA Office of Pollution Prevention and Toxics	www.epa.gov/aboutepa/about-office-chemical-safety-and-pollution-prevention-ocspp#oppt Chemicals under the Toxic Substances Control Act (TSCA): www.epa.gov/opptintr/index TSCA Hotline: 1-202-554-1404
– US EPA Toxics Release Inventory Program	www.epa.gov/toxics-release-inventory-tri-program
– US EPA *America's Children and the Environment*	www.epa.gov/americaschildrenenvironment
– US EPA Sun Safety	www.epa.gov/sunsafety
– US EPA "Health Research Grants"	www.epa.gov/research-grants/health-research-grants

US Food and Drug Administration (FDA) 10903 New Hampshire Ave Silver Spring, MD 20993	www.fda.gov 1-888-INFO-FDA (1-888-463-6332)
– Center for Food Safety and Applied Nutrition (CFSAN) 5001 Campus Drive # HFS-009 College Park, MD 20740-3835	www.fda.gov/about-fda/fda-organization/center-food-safety-and-applied-nutrition-cfsan 1-888-SAFEFOOD (1-888-723-3366)
– Foodsafety.gov: Your Gateway to Federal Food Safety Information	www.foodsafety.gov
– Center for Tobacco Products (CTP) US Food and Drug Administration (FDA) 10903 New Hampshire Ave Document Control Center Bldg 71, Room G335 Silver Spring, MD 20993-0002	www.fda.gov/tobacco-products
US Global Change Research Program 1800 G St NW Ste 9100 Washington, DC 20006	www.globalchange.gov

Organization	Contact Information
STATE AGENCIES	
California Environmental Protection Agency	www.calepa.ca.gov
New York State Children's Environmental Health Centers	www.nyscheck.org
US Environmental Protection Agency (EPA) list of state health and environmental agencies with links to websites	www.epa.gov/home/health-and-environmental-agencies-us-states-and-territories
NON-US GOVERNMENTS	
Canadian Partnership for Children's Health and Environment c/o 1500-55 University Avenue Toronto, ON M5J 2H7 Canada	www.healthyenvironmentforkids.ca
European Union information on environmental health	www.europa.eu/european-union/topics/environment_en

Intergovernmental Panel on Climate Change (IPCC)	www.ipcc.ch
Registration, Evaluation, Authorisation and Restriction of Chemicals (REACH)	www.ec.europa.eu/environment/chemicals/reach/reach_en.htm
World Health Organization (WHO) Public Health, Environmental and Social Determinants of Health	www.who.int/phe/en
– Healthy Environments for Children Alliance	www.who.int/heca/en
– Global Initiative on Children's Environmental Health Indicators	www.who.int/ceh/indicators/en
– Children's Environmental Health	www.who.int/ceh/en
– Training Package for Health Care Providers	www.who.int/ceh/capacity/trainpackage/en
– WHO Collaborating Centres for Children's Environmental Health	"Working Together: WHO Collaborating Centres for Children's Environmental Health": www.who.int/ceh/ceh_ccnetwork/en
– WHO Water Sanitation Hygiene	www.who.int/water_sanitation_health/en
– WHO information about chemical safety	www.who.int/pcs
– WHO information about radiation	www.who.int/ionizing_radiation/en

Organization	Contact Information
World Health Organization (WHO) Public Health, Environmental and Social Determinants of Health (*continued*)	
– WHO information about air pollution	www.who.int/health-topics/air-pollution#tab=tab_1
– WHO information about ultraviolet radiation	www.who.int/peh-uv
– WHO information about electromagnetic fields	www.who.int/peh-emf/en
– WHO information about occupational health	www.who.int/oeh/index.html
NONGOVERNMENTAL ORGANIZATIONS	
Allergy & Asthma Network 8229 Boone Blvd Ste 260 Vienna, VA 22182	www.allergyasthmanetwork.org 1-800-878-4403
Alliance for Healthy Homes 227 Massachusetts Ave NE Ste 200 Washington, DC 20002	www.afhh.org 1-202-543-1147
American Academy of Pediatrics 345 Park Blvd Itasca, IL 60143	www.aap.org 1-800-433-9016

American Association of Poison Control Centers 4601 North Fairfax Dr Ste 630 Arlington, VA 22203	www.aapcc.org Poison Control Center: 1-800-222-1222
American Cancer Society 250 Williams St NW Atlanta, GA 30303	www.cancer.org 1-800-ACS-2345 (1-800-227-2345)
American Lung Association 55 W Wacker Dr Ste 1150 Chicago, IL 60601	www.lung.org 1-800-LUNGUSA (1-800-586-4872)
Asthma and Allergy Foundation of America 1235 S Clark St Ste 305 Arlington, VA 22202	www.aafa.org 1-800-7-ASTHMA (1-800-727-8462)
Beyond Pesticides 701 E St SE Ste 200 Washington, DC 20003	www.beyondpesticides.org info@beyondpesticides.org 1-202-543-5450

Organization	Contact Information
Birth Defects Research and Prevention 11190 Sunrise Valley Dr Ste 300 Reston, VA 20191-4375	birthdefectsresearch.org bdrp@birthdefectsresearch.org 1-703-438-3104
Center for Health, Environment and Justice 7139 Shreve Rd Falls Church, VA 22046 PO Box 6806 Falls Church, VA 22040	www.chej.org info@chej.org 1-703-237-2249
Children's Environmental Health and Disease Prevention Research Centers	www.niehs.nih.gov/research/supported/centers/prevention/grantees/index.cfm
– Children's Environmental Health and Disease Prevention Center at Dartmouth	www.dartmouth.edu/~childrenshealth
– Columbia University Mailman School of Public Health	www.mailman.columbia.edu
– Duke University Neurodevelopment and Improving Children's Health following Environmental Tobacco Smoke exposure (NICHES)	www.niehs.nih.gov/research/supported/centers/prevention/grantees/duke/index.cfm

− Emory University Center for Children's Health, the Environment, the Microbiome, and Metabolomics (C-CHEM²)	www.nursing.emory.edu/c-chem2/index.html
− Johns Hopkins University	www.niehs.nih.gov/research/supported/centers/prevention/grantees/johns-hopkins/index.cfm
− National Jewish Health Environmental Determinants of Airway Disease in Children	www.epa.gov/research-grants/niehsepa-cehcs-denver-childrens-environmental-health-center-environmental
− Northeastern University Center for Research on Early Childhood Exposure and Development in Puerto Rico (CRECE)	www.northeastern.edu/crece
− Southern California Children's Environmental Health Center (SC-CEHC)	www.niehs.nih.gov/research/supported/centers/prevention/grantees/usc/index.cfm
− University of California, Davis, Center for Children's Environmental Health and Disease Prevention	www.ucdmc.ucdavis.edu/mindinstitute/research/cceh/index.html
− University of California at Berkeley Center for Environmental Research and Children's Health (CERCH)	cerch.berkeley.edu/home

Organization	Contact Information
Children's Environmental Health and Disease Prevention Research Centers (*continued*)	
– University of California at Berkeley Center for Integrative Research on Childhood Leukemia and the Environment	circle.berkeley.edu www.niehs.nih.gov/research/supported/centers/prevention/grantees/berkeley-circle/index.cfm
– University of California San Francisco Pregnancy Exposures to Environmental Chemicals (PEEC) Children's Center	prhe.ucsf.edu/childrens-center
– University of Michigan Children's Environmental Health and Disease Prevention Research Center	sph.umich.edu/cehc
Children's Environmental Health Network 110 Maryland Ave NE Ste 404 Washington, DC 20002	cehn.org cehn@cehn.org 1-202-543-4033
Children's Environmental Health Institute PO Box 50342 Austin, TX 78763-0342	cehi.org 1-512-657-7405

Commonweal 451 Mesa Rd (PO Box 316 for post office mail) Bolinas, CA 94924	www.commonweal.org 1-415-868-0970
Earth Portal	www.earthportal.org
EMR Network PO Box 1440 Montpelier, VT 05601	emrnetwork.org info@emrnetwork.org
Environmental Defense Fund 257 Park Ave S New York, NY 10010	www.edf.org 1-202-572-3298
Environmental Working Group 1436 U St NW Ste 100 Washington, DC 20009	www.ewg.org 1-202-667-6982
Health Care Without Harm 12355 Sunrise Valley Dr Ste 680 Reston, VA 20191	noharm.org info@hcwh.org 1-703-860-9790

Organization	Contact Information
Healthy Schools Network 153 Regent St Ste 1050 Saratoga Springs, NY 12866	www.healthyschools.org info@healthyschools.org 1-518-462-0632
Institute for Agriculture and Trade Policy 2105 1st Ave S Minneapolis, MN 55404	www.iatp.org info@iatp.org 1-612-870-0453
International Research and Information Network on Children's Health, Environment and Safety	inchesnetwork.net info@inchesnetwork.net
International Society for Children's Health & the Environment	ische.ca
Learning Disabilities Association of America 461 Cochran Rd Ste 245 Pittsburgh, PA 15228	ldaamerica.org info@ldaamerica.org 1-412-341-1515
March of Dimes Foundation 1550 Crystal Dr Ste 1300 Arlington, VA 22202	www.marchofdimes.org 1-888-MODIMES (1-888-663-4637)

Moms Clean Air Force	www.momscleanairforce.org
National Center for Healthy Housing 10320 Little Patuxent Pkwy Ste 500 Columbia, MD 21044	nchh.org 1-410-992-0712
National Council on Skin Cancer Prevention	skincancerprevention.org
National Environmental Education Foundation 4301 Connecticut Ave NW Ste 160 Washington, DC 20008-2326	www.neefusa.org 1-202-833-2933
National Lead Information Center 422 S Clinton Ave Rochester, NY 14620	www.epa.gov/lead/nlic.htm 1-800-424-LEAD (1-800-424-5323)
National Pesticide Information Center Oregon State University 310 Weniger Hall Corvallis, OR 97331-6502	npic.orst.edu npic@ace.orst.edu 1-800-858-7378
National Safety Council "Indoor Air: The Good and the Bad"	www.nsc.org/home-safety/safety-topics/other-poisons/air-quality

Organization	Contact Information
National School Integrated Pest Management Information Sources	schoolipm.ifas.ufl.edu
Natural Resources Defense Council 40 W 20th St 11th Floor New York, NY 10011	www.nrdc.org rdcinfo@nrdc.org 1-212-727-2700
Our Stolen Future	www.ourstolenfuture.com
Pediatric Environmental Health Specialty Units (PEHSUs)	www.pehsu.net (Includes links to all PEHSUs)
New England PEHSU—Boston, MA *Academic Affiliation:* Harvard Medical School and Harvard School of Public Health *Hospital Affiliation:* Boston Children's Hospital and Cambridge Hospital **Connecticut, Maine, Massachusetts, New Hampshire, Rhode Island, and Vermont**	www.childrenshospital.org/pehc 1-617-355-8177 or 1-888-CHILD14 (1-888-244-5314)

PEHSU—New York, NY *Academic Affiliation:* Icahn School of Medicine at Mount Sinai Department of Preventive Medicine *Hospital Affiliation:* The Mount Sinai Hospital **New Jersey, New York, Puerto Rico, and US Virgin Islands**	icahn.mssm.edu/research/pehsu pehsu@mssm.edu 1-866-265-6201
Mid-Atlantic Center for Children's Health and the Environment PEHSU—Washington, DC *Academic Affiliation:* Georgetown University *Hospital Affiliation:* Georgetown University Medical Center **Delaware; Maryland; Pennsylvania; Virginia; Washington, DC; and West Virginia**	kidsandenvironment.georgetown.edu kidsandenvironment@georgetown.edu 1-866-622-2431
Southeast PEHSU—Atlanta, GA *Academic Affiliation:* Emory University Department of Pediatrics *Hospital Affiliation:* Children's Healthcare of Atlanta—Egleston Children's Hospital and Hughes Spalding Children's Hospital **Alabama, Florida, Georgia, Kentucky, Mississippi, North Carolina, South Carolina, and Tennessee**	www.pediatrics.emory.edu/centers/pehsu/index.html www.pehsu.net/region4.html 1-404-727-9428 1-877-33-PEHSU (1-877-337-3478)

Organization	Contact Information
Pediatric Environmental Health Specialty Units (PEHSUs) *(continued)*	
Great Lakes Center PEHSU—Chicago, IL *Academic Affiliation:* University of Illinois at Chicago School of Public Health *Hospital Affiliation:* Stroger Hospital of Cook County **Illinois, Indiana, Michigan, Minnesota, Ohio, and Wisconsin**	great-lakes.uic.edu/childrens-environmental-health childrensenviro@uic.edu 1-312-864-5526 1-866-967-7337
Southwest Center for Pediatric Environmental Health PEHSU—El Paso, TX *Academic Affiliation:* Texas Tech University Health Sciences Center Paul L. Foster School of Medicine *Hospital Affiliation:* University Medical Center of El Paso and El Paso Children's Hospital **Arkansas, Louisiana, New Mexico, Oklahoma, and Texas**	swcpeh.org swcpeh@ttuhsc.edu 1-915-534-3807 1-888-901-5665

Mid-America PEHSU—Kansas City, MO *Academic Affiliation:* University of Missouri-Kansas City School of Medicine *Hospital Affiliation:* Children's Mercy Hospitals and Clinics **Iowa, Kansas, Missouri, and Nebraska**	www.childrensmercy.org/mapehsu mapehsu@cmh.edu 1-913-588-6638 1-800-421-9916
Rocky Mountain Region PEHSU—Denver, CO *Academic Affiliation:* University of Colorado Health Sciences Center *Hospital Affiliation:* Denver Health and Hospitals Authority and the Rocky Mountain Poison and Drug Center **Colorado, Montana, North Dakota, South Dakota, Utah, and Wyoming**	www.denverhealth.org/services/community-health/pediatric-environmental-health-specialty-unit 1-877-800-5554

Organization	Contact Information
Pediatric Environmental Health Specialty Units (PEHSUs) *(continued)*	
Western States PEHSU—San Francisco, CA *Academic Affiliation:* University of California San Francisco *Hospital Affiliation:* University of California San Francisco Medical Center **Arizona, California, Hawaii, and Nevada**	wspehsu.ucsf.edu pehsu@ucsf.edu 1-415-514-0878 1-866-UC-PEHSU (1-866-827-3478)
Northwest PEHSU—Seattle, WA *Academic Affiliation:* University of Washington: Department of Occupational and Environmental Health Sciences, Occupational and Environmental Medicine program, and Department of Pediatrics *Hospital Affiliation:* University of Washington Medical Center, Harborview Medical Center, and Seattle Children's Hospital **Alaska, Idaho, Oregon, and Washington**	deohs.washington.edu/pehsu/about-us pehsu@uw.edu 1-877-KID-CHEM (1-877-543-2436)

Physicians for Social Responsibility 1111 14th St NW Ste 700 Washington, DC 20005	www.psr.org psrnatl@psr.org 1-202-667-4260
– Pediatric Environmental Health Toolkit	peht.ucsf.edu
Shopper's Guide to Pesticides in Produce	www.ewg.org/foodnews
Smoke Free Home	www.kidslivesmokefree.org

Index

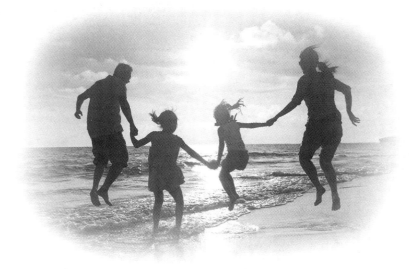

Index

About the Editors

Editor in Chief: Ruth A. Etzel, MD, PhD, FAAP

Dr Etzel is an internationally recognized pediatrician, environmental epidemiologist, and preventive medicine specialist. She performed the first study to document that children with secondhand exposure to tobacco smoke had measurable exposure to nicotine. Her pioneering work led to nationwide efforts to reduce indoor exposure to tobacco, including the ban on smoking in US airliners. She also produced the first research to show that exposure to toxigenic molds in the home could be dangerous to infant health. She served on the American Academy of Pediatrics Committee on Environmental Health from 1986 to 1995 and chaired it from 1995 to 1999. From 2009 to 2012, she led the World Health Organization activities to protect children from environmental hazards. Dr Etzel is the editor of *Pediatric Environmental Health*.

Associate Editor: Sophie J. Balk, MD, FAAP

Dr Balk is a general pediatrician at The Children's Hospital at Montefiore and professor of pediatrics at the Albert Einstein College of Medicine in Bronx, NY. Her academic work focuses on educating clinicians about pediatric environmental health. She is a current member and past chair of the American Academy of Pediatrics Council on Environmental Health Executive Committee and a past member of the American Academy of Pediatrics Section on Tobacco Control Executive Committee. She has served as associate editor of the 4 editions of *Pediatric Environmental Health*. Dr Balk has published and lectured on skin cancer prevention, tobacco issues, noise exposure, and other environmental health issues relevant to pediatric practice.